Gender and Recovery
from Coronary Artery Bypass Surgery

A Psychological Perspective

# Fortschritte der Herz-, Thorax-und Gefäßchirurgie

Herausgegeben von R. Hetzer

## Band 7

Friederike Kendel

# Gender and Recovery from Coronary Artery Bypass Surgery

A Psychological Perspective

Steinkopff Verlag

Dr. FRIEDERIKE KENDEL, Dipl.-Psych.
Wissenschaftliche Mitarbeiterin
Institut für Medizinische Psychologie
Luisenstraße 57
10117 Berlin

ISBN 978-3-7985-1855-1 Steinkopff Verlag

Cataloging-in-Publication Data applied for
A catalog record for this book is available from the Library of Congress.
Bibliographic information published by Die Deutsche Bibliothek
Die Deutsche Bibliothek lists this publication in the Deutsche Nationalbibliografie;
detailed bibliographic data is available in the Internet at http://dnb.d-nb.de.

Steinkopff Verlag
a member of Springer Science+Business Media

www.steinkopff.com

© Steinkopff Verlag 2009
  Printed in Germany

The use of general descriptive names, registered names, trademarks, etc. in this publication does not imply, even in the absence of a specific statement, that such names are exempt from the relevant protective laws and regulations and therefore free for general use.

Product liability: The publishers cannot guarantee the accuracy of any information about the application of operative techniques and medications contained in this book. In every individual case the user must check such information by consulting the relevant literature.

SPIN 12539161       85/7231-5  4  3  2  1  0 – Printed on acid-free paper

# Foreword

Progress in coronary artery bypass graft surgery has irrefutably improved the quality of life of many patients. However, we are confronted with the finding that women exhibit a higher mortality rate than men. In part, this difference can be explained by clinical parameters such as age, disease severity, or comorbidity – factors that have been well studied, but which do not fully explain the observed differences. This is one reason why, in recent years, psychosocial variables have attracted special attention in this context. In fact, women and men having undergone a bypass operation vary a great deal with respect to, e.g., depression, partner status, and socio-economic status. Moreover, psychological well-being, on the one hand, and social isolation, on the other hand, definitely influence the recovery process, particularly when considered under the gender aspect.

The *Deutsches Herzzentrum Berlin* has been actively supporting gender-specific research for many years. In this context, a large prospective study on gender differences in recovery after bypass surgery, carried out by the Competence Network of Heart Failure, was started at our Department for Cardiothoracic and Vascular Surgery. From the beginning of the study, psychosocial variables were included as being substantial contributors.

The starting point of the study presented here* by psychologist Dr. Friederike Kendel are recent empirical investigations about gender differences in coronary heart disease and the course of recovery after bypass surgery. On this basis, depression, social support, and specific stress factors from a gender point of view are carefully evaluated over a one-year period (starting a few days before operation). In order to measure the effect of these factors not only the mortality rate is evaluated, but the present study also focuses on the patients' subjectively perceived quality of life.

This treatise fills an important gap in cardiovascular research. Using an interdisciplinary approach, psychosocial findings are presented within a framework of medical parameters. The often so tiring statistical analyses are explained with clarity, wherever possible in words comprehensible also for non-statisticians. Thus, the book is addressed not only to psychologists, but also to medical students, cardiologists, or general physicians, who are interested in the upcoming field of Medical Psychology.

Prof. Roland Hetzer
Chairman, German Heart Institute Berlin

---

* Based on the thesis in Medical Psychology at Charité – Universitätsmedizin Berlin by Friederike Kendel "Gender Differences in Mortality and Physical Functioning After Coronary Artery Bypass Graft Surgery: An Analysis from a Psychosocial Perspective"

# CONTENTS

# 1 INTRODUCTION

Coronary artery bypass graft (CABG) surgery is an outstanding example for the tremendous technological and demographic changes that have taken place during the past five decades. Today, about 100 000 CABG operations are performed annually in Germany, of which roughly 25% are on women (StBA, 2007). The operation is performed to relieve angina pectoris and to reduce the risk of death from coronary heart disease (CHD). In order to bypass atherosclerotic narrowing, either veins from the leg or the left internal mammary artery are grafted from the aorta to the coronary arteries. Thereby the impaired blood supply of the heart is improved. From a medical point of view, differences in body surface area are related to a difference in vessel size. Because smaller coronary arteries may be more difficult to operate on, some authors have suggested that complete revascularization may be harder to achieve for women compared to men (Osswald et al., 2001; Humphries et al., 2007). Complications that can occur after surgery are, amongst others, infections at incision sites, deep vein thrombosis, malunion of the sternum, stroke during reperfusion, chronic pain at incision sites and postoperative stress-related illnesses. Of all patients, 3-4% die in the first 28 days after surgery, a time span, which is referred to as early mortality or in-hospital mortality, respectively. Gender differences in the early mortality rate have been the object of intense debate in numerous studies.

After this short glimpse at the procedure, a description of gender differences in mortality rates will be given. Subsequently, risk factors are elaborated in detail, differentiating between somatic and psychosocial factors. Finally, outcome parameters such as quality of life and depression are discussed with respect to gender. Throughout the present study, the term "gender" encompasses both biological sex and gender in its actual sense.

## 1.1 Gender Differences in Mortality after CABG

Vaccarino et al. (2002) stated that women tend to have higher early mortality rates than men in all age groups. However, the risk was considerably higher among younger women and was only partially accounted for by differences in comorbid conditions and cardiovascular risk factors. Blankstein et al. (2005) found that, even after adjustment for all identifiable risk factors, women undergoing CABG continued to have a higher early mortality than men. While women appeared to have a mortality rate that was 90% higher than their male counterparts, after risk adjustment this gender gap in early mortality decreased to 22%. Other researchers could not confirm these results. Toumpoulis et al. (2006) found no differences in early mortality after adjustment for clinical risk factors. Rather female sex was an independent predictor of improved 5-year survival rate.

The first detailed analysis in a large European cohort on the interaction of sex and age in early mortality was provided by Regitz-Zagrosek et al. (2004). In the younger age cohort (< 70.5 years) there was a significant impact of gender on mortality, which diminished with increasing age and did not reach significance in the older age cohort. In this study, too, the gender difference with respect to mortality remained significant after adjustment for conventional risk factors. A summary of studies explicitly addressing gender differences in early mortality is given in Table 1.

**Table 1. Gender Differences in Early Mortality After CABG**

| Reference | N | Women | RR[1] (Women vs. Men) | Female gender as a risk factor after adjustment for clinical risk factors |
|---|---|---|---|---|
| Bestawros et al. (2005) | 12 017 | 24% | 1.67 | Female gender significant |
| Blankstein et al. (2005) | 15 440 | 33% | 1.90 | Female gender significant |
| Regitz-Zagrosek et al. (2004) | 17 528 | 24% | 1.51 | Female gender significant in age group<70.5 years |
| Vaccarino et al. (2002) | 51 187 | 30% | 1.83 | Female gender significant in age group<50 years |
| Abramov et al. (2000) | 4 823 | 19% | 1.50 | Female gender not significant |
| Edwards (1998) | 344 913 | 28% | 1.73 | Female gender in the entire sample significant. but not in high-risk patients |
| Bandrup-Wogensen (1996) | 2 129 | 19% | 2.50 | Female gender significant |

Note. (1) Risk Ratios

Female gender has been listed as a risk factor for adverse outcome after cardiac surgery in the EuroSCORE algorithm, which is a well-established and validated model for contemporary practice in cardiac surgery (Nashef et al., 1999). Over the past years, however, there has been increasing evidence that the gender difference in mortality is narrowing. Humphries et al. (2007) reported that the in-hospital mortality in women improved significantly between 1991 and 2004, declining from 5.6 to 1.9%. Despite this improvement, women were still 42% more likely to die within this time period than men. Other research groups have reported similar results (O'Rourke et al., 2001, Ghali et al., 2003).

In this context, the question arises whether the gender difference in outcome persists after all identifiable risk factors have been accounted for. In other words: is female sex simply a marker of a high-risk profile? And what role do psychosocial factors play?

Women generally exhibit a higher early mortality rate after CABG than men. Additionally, some studies have shown an interaction between gender and age, with younger women having higher mortality rates. Women's excess in mortality is attributable, but only to a limited extent, to identifiable gender differences in baseline health status. The cause of the remaining difference is unknown as yet.

## 1.2   Gender Aspects of Risk Factors

Risk factors that contribute to coronary heart disease (CHD) also influence the course after bypass surgery. Therefore this section addresses the epidemiology of CHD, its development and the main cardiovascular risk factors, with the main focus on studies considering gender.

For several decades now, cardiovascular disease – and CHD in particular – has been the leading cause of death in Western industrialized nations. CHD is the result of an accumulation of atheromatous plaques on the walls of the arteries that supply the myocardium with oxygen. The vast majority of research on CHD in Germany to date has been conducted almost exclusively in male populations (see Mittag, 2002). The findings of these studies have frequently been extrapolated to women, despite the fact that there are a variety of biological differences between men and women that make such a generalization highly questionable. It has been known for some time that there are gender-specific differences in risk factor profiles, as well as in symptom manifestation and issues related to starting and managing therapies. Nonetheless, gender differences in cardiovascular risks did not become an important focus of research on an international scale until the early 1990s. In the following sections, risk factors that play a role in the development and the course of CHD will be described.

### 1.2.1   Somatic Risk Factors

Data on the prevalence of risk factors represent an important basis for estimating the relative risk of developing CHD. Modifiable risk factors comprise smoking, overweight, diabetes and high cholesterol levels as well as lack of exercise, elevated lipoprotein levels and psychosocial factors. The INTERHEART-study (Yusuf et al., 2004) described and quantified the main risk factors for CHD in detail for 52 countries. According to these analyses, smoking, high lipid concentrations and stress are the main risk factors for coronary artery disease worldwide. Besides diabetes, hypertension and the pattern of fat distribution (waist to hip ratio) play an important role in pathophysiology. Moderate consumption of alcohol, physical activity and a balanced diet are seen as protective factors.

However, there are striking gender- and age-related differences in risk factor profiles among individuals. Therefore, individual risk factors will be described in detail with respect to their gender aspects.

**Smoking**

Cigarette smoking is the most important single risk factor for the development of CHD in women and men. In the early 1980s it was already becoming clear that in Germany smoking and oral contraceptive use were the two risk factors in younger female patients (< 50) that were tied to issues of social status as well as family and career planning (Weidemann et al., 2003). Between 1983 and 2003 the number of women smokers steadily increased, whereas the opposite is true for men. Among women aged 25 to 69 the smoking rate increased from 27% to 30%. In contrast, smoking among men over the same period showed a decline from 42% to 38%. Studies conducted in the 1980s show that smoking among women is often associated with emotional stress, whether this be related to work and/or other psychosocial burdens (Weidemann et al, 2003). As a risk factor for CHD, smoking appears to be particularly harmful to women. In one study, current female smokers had a relative risk for myocardial infarction of 2.2 compared with female non-smokers; for male smokers, however, the relative risk was 1.4 (Prescott et al., 1998). Active smoking is associated with a drastic reduction in the age of onset for first myocardial infarction: in one study, the average age reduction was 19 years for women (from 79 to 60 years of age) and 7 years for men (from 71 to 64) (Hansen et al., 1993).

**Hypertension**

Smoking plays a less important role in the cardiovascular risk profile of older women, which is characterized by a combination of hypertension, overweight and diabetes (Weidemann et al., 2003). The prevalence of hypertension in both men and women increases steadily with advancing age. Until the age of 60, the prevalence of hypertension is higher in men than in women, but this is reversed in older age groups (Rich-Edwards et al., 1995). Prospective epidemiological studies have consistently shown that hypertension increases the cardiovascular risk for men and women: approximately 60% of the cases of heart failure and half of the cases of myocardial infarction are linked to hypertension (Park et al., 2003). Findings from the Framingham Study indicated that hypertension increased the age and risk factor adjusted hazard of heart failure twofold in men and threefold in women (Kannel, 2000).

**Cholesterol**

In most populations the cholesterol levels increase with age. In men this increase reaches its peak level at the age of 45-50 years, whereas in women the increase does not stop before the age of

60-65 years (Jousilahti et al., 1996). It has long been known that in men an increase in cholesterol of 1% is associated with an increase in risk for CHD of 2-3% (LaRosa et al., 1990). Moreover, in a meta-analysis of 86 000 women high levels of total and LDL cholesterol were strong predictors of CHD mortality in women under 65 years of age (Walsh and Grady, 1995). In the Framingham study the 16-year incidence increased continuously with the ratio of total cholesterol to HDL cholesterol. However, this increase was steeper for women than for men (Kannel and Wilson, 1995).

**Diabetes**

Diabetes is another risk factor that bears more serious complications for women than for men in the context of CHD. If suffering from diabetes, women seem to lose the protection normally afforded them by oestrogen in younger age groups (Härtel, 2003). Indeed, diabetes increases the risk of myocardial infarction sixfold in women and only fourfold in men (Löwel et al., 1999). Diabetes also increases the early mortality after a myocardial infarction: 18% for women, but only 9.9% for men (Löwel et al., 2000).

**Body Mass Index**

Obesity is usually defined in terms of "body mass index" (BMI). The BMI is calculated by dividing one's weight (in kilograms) by the square of one's height (in m). The WHO defined overweight as a BMI of 25 to 29.9 and obesity as a BMI of 30 or greater. The patterns of lipid accumulation differ between women and men. Premenopausal women more frequently develop peripheral obesity with subcutaneous fat accumulation, whereas men and postmenopausal women are more prone to central or android obesity (Regitz-Zagrosek et al., 2006). Obesity raises cardiovascular risks partly through its effects on established risk factors such as hypertension, dyslipidemia, glucose intolerance and insulin resistance (Rexrode et al., 1996). Many long-term prospective studies have shown a strong association between being overweight and CHD, which appears to be linear. Epidemiological studies have generally demonstrated stronger associations between overweight and CHD in women than in men (Rexrode et al., 2001). The causes for this difference are still unclear. The elevated risk ratio in women may be partly due to their lower baseline risk of CHD compared to men (Haffner et al., 1991).

Known risk factors for CHD in men obviously also apply to women. However, comparing the prevalence of risk factors in women and men is of only limited value, since several risk factors constitute a different relative risk of CHD, beyond their varying impact in different age groups. In particular, smoking, diabetes, hypertension, high cholesterol levels and a high BMI represent a considerably higher coronary risk for women than for men.

### 1.2.2 Psychosocial Risk Factors

Over the past several years, a growing body of evidence has made clear that not only somatic, but also psychosocial risk factors play a role in the development and clinical manifestation of coronary heart disease. Psychosocial and biological factors often influence each other in a reciprocal manner, and somatic risk factors such as smoking, overweight, or hypercholesterolemia are often the result of lifestyle behaviour developed in response to stressful life events. In the INTERHEART study (N = 15 000) (Yusuf et al., 2004) psychosocial risk factors, which are known to be associated with an increased risk for myocardial infarction (MI) were analyzed carefully. Worldwide, the relation between stress and an increased MI risk has been demonstrated (Yusuf et al., 2004; Orth-Gomer et al., 2000; Stone, 1999) and appears to be consistent over all regions. Stress was accountable for 22% of MIs (Yusuf et al., 2004). However, stress was assessed retrospectively and on the basis of only four items. Like all retrospective studies of subjective factors, this carries the risk that subsequent events may distort memory. In the context of CHD, depression and a lack of social support have gained significance over the last years. In contrast, after an extensive meta-analysis provided by Myrtek (2001) concerning the influence of type-A-behaviour on CHD, it is assumed that the type-A construct has become less relevant (see Knoll et al., 2005).

In the following the psychosocial risk factors will be described with regard to their relevance for CHD. Gender-differentiating findings will be added where reported.

### Depression as a Risk Factor

Depression is a common comorbid condition in coronary heart disease. Frequently, depressive moods are prodromal to an infarction, although it is not always possible to diagnose these in an objective manner. Such "premanifest" illness behaviour, characterized by energy loss and exhaustion, may be relatively non-specific. The question as to whether these factors independently influence the course of disease is still largely unexplored (Ladwig et al., 2004). Depression is associated with a number of behavioural risk factors, such as smoking, alcohol abuse and physical inactivity. On a physiological level, these behaviours correspond, for example, with overweight, diabetes and hypertension. Unhealthy behaviour, a lack of care and financial restraints are typically associated with hopelessness and an increased mortality. Chronic stress has frequently been cited as a behavioural, and thus modifiable, risk factor in men and women alike. However, in contrast to the most frequently investigated somatic risk factors, elucidating the exact role played by stress in MI has been difficult. This may be due to the fact that insufficient attention has been paid to the affective manifestations of chronic emotional distress, such as feelings of "burn-out", exhaustion, or pessimism about the future – all of which can contribute to depression or depressive moods (Ladwig et al., 2004).

Frasure-Smith et al. (1999) studied the risk of mortality in hospitalized MI patients, with 1-year follow-up. Of the depressed women in this sample, 8.3% died during the follow-up year in contrast to 7% of men diagnosed as depressive. Controlling for previous MI, left ventricular ejection fraction (LVEF) and smoking did not change the influence of depression on mortality significantly. Therefore, depression is an independent predictor for 1-year cardiac mortality and is largely independent of other risk factors. In previous investigations depression was found to have a greater impact on poor cardiovascular outcome in women than in men (Williams et al., 2002; Mendes de Leon et al., 1998). This suggests a greater vulnerability of women not only towards depression, which is well established, but also towards the adverse effects of depression on the cardiovascular system.

The relationship between depression and mortality after MI or bypass surgery has become more and more evident (Barefoot et al., 1996, Blumenthal et al., 2003). Depression either before or after surgery is associated with a worse outcome in terms of rehospitalization in the first postoperative weeks (Saur et al., 2001) as well as mortality in the years after surgery. However, the reasons remained unclear. In a study by Burg et al. (2003) of male CABG patients, 24% of the depressed men had been rehospitalized in the first 6 weeks after surgery in contrast to only 3% of the non-depressive patients. The influence of depression proved to be independent of a series of clinical and operation-specific indices that also relate to morbidity after CABG. Another finding of this study was the influence of preoperative depression on quality of life after discharge from hospital. Men diagnosed with depression reported more pain and the probability of them returning to their prior level of functioning was reduced. Mallik et al. (2005) confirmed these results. They found a close relationship between the number of depressive symptoms at baseline and improvement after surgery in physical functioning. In multivariate analysis depression tended to be an even stronger inverse risk factor for functional improvement after CABG than traditional measures of disease severity such as history of myocardial infarction, diabetes or congestive heart failure. The inverse association between depressive symptoms and improvement in functional status was stronger in women than in men.

Connerney et al. (2001) conducted structured psychiatric interviews with CABG patients before their discharge from hospital and repeated the interview 1 year later. In the group of depressed patients, 27% had had a cardiac event at 12 months compared to 10% who were not depressed. Female sex had a positive univariate association with cardiac outcomes after discharge from hospital. However, depression was not a predictor of mortality or non-cardiac events in this setting. Since the mortality rate in relation to the whole number of bypass operations is relatively small, the non-significant relationship between depression and mortality could be ascribed to a lack of power in these studies. Blumenthal et al. (2003) therefore conducted a longitudinal study of 817 patients, who were followed-up for up to 12 years. Patients with moderate to severe depression at baseline had higher rates of death than those without depression. The influence of depression was independent of other risk factors. This study had several methodological limitations. First, medical data were collected only before surgery, which did not allow assessment of how changes in cardiac function during the follow-up could have affected symptoms of depression postoperatively. Second, the data analysis was not differentiated by gender, so that gender-specific information is lacking.

**Anxiety**

High levels of anxiety often accompany the wait for surgery. The degree of anxiety is important because too little or too much anxiety interferes with postoperative recovery whereas moderate anxiety improves coping with the situation (Koivula et al., 2001). Moderate levels of anxiety can help patients to adequately prepare for surgery and reduce stress. Whereas anxiety is more common before surgery and is associated with the threat of the surgical procedure itself, depressive symptoms are likely to predominate in the time period after surgery. However, the difficulties with the resumption of household tasks and social demands after CABG experienced by a vast majority of patients can lead to anxiety postoperatively as well (Underwood et al., 1993). As anxiety and depression are interrelated, higher levels of anxiety may be associated with higher levels of depression.

**Socioeconomic Status**

For both men and women, low socioeconomic status is associated with lifestyle behaviours that increase one's susceptibility to cardiac disease: heavy smoking, increased stress, unhealthy eating habits and physical inactivity (Brezinka and Kittel, 1996).

In the Stanford Five-City Project, for both genders higher cholesterol levels, higher hypertension rates, more smoking and higher BMI were associated with a lower education level (Winkleby et al., 1990). This association remained highly significant after adjustment for income and profession. Each increase in educational level corresponded with a decrease in the total risk score. However, socioeconomic status appeared to have a stronger effect on women with regard to cardiac mortality than it did on men. For women a low socioeconomic status often means being economically dependent. This substantially restricts one's actions and access to other resources. Often, if women are not gainfully employed, the social network is their main resource and work in the home is their main focus. But the social network of women is often demanding and supportive at the same time and, indeed, a majority of studies show that women perceive themselves as receiving less support than do men.

**Social Support**

Interpersonal relationships may help to obtain additional resources and to preserve them. This is true for material goods, but also for immaterial goods such as emotional support and affection. The latter resources gain particular importance in times of crises, when basic personal resources such as health, socioeconomic status or well-being are endangered (Hobfoll and Wells, 1998). Social support, in particular, is an important resource in coping with stress.

Social support has a wide variety of meanings. The construct can be split into a qualitative and quantitative dimension. The quantitative dimension is referred to as social integration. To measure social integration, structural and quantitative aspects are considered, such as network size or frequency of interactions (Rieckmann, 2003). In contrast, the qualitative dimension refers to the functional and qualitative support provided by others. This dimension of social support can be provided in terms of emotional support or instrumental support (Berkman and Glass, 2000).

Men and women differ with regard to their network sizes. Women, when asked about their number of close relationships, generally had a larger social network (Pugliesi and Shook, 1998). Usually they provide more social support than men do, and, in return, seem to receive more (Laireiter and Baumann, 1992). Women of all ages are more likely than men to turn to others for support in times of adverse life events. They usually possess a larger social network, which is, however, linked with costs. Men seem to rely on fewer ties, but benefit more from those. In married couples, they are more likely than women to name their spouse as a primary confidant (Berkman et al., 1993). Seeking support outside the marriage is less likely for men and has been shown to be associated with an increase in depression (Edwards et al., 1998).

Social isolation and lack of support increases the probability of cardiac events (Schwarzer and Rieckmann, 2002). Even a short time after the cardiac event, social support is an important predictor for recovery. Kulik and Mahler (1989) measured the length of hospitalization of male CHD patients with and without a partner. Patients without a partner and with low social support were hospitalized for longer than patients with a partner and more social support. Few studies, however, have investigated the association between social support and health-related quality of life after bypass surgery. These studies have yielded conflicting results. Some have shown beneficial influences of both emotional or instrumental support (Oxman and Hull, 1997), while others did not show any relationship between emotional support and quality of life, but rather between instrumental support and quality of life (Elizur and Hirsh, 1999).

## Role of Partner Status

If marriage were a measure of social support, men and women would be expected to benefit equally from it. Generally, married people rank their health higher and feel less lonely. But these effects are, in an intercultural comparison, stronger for married men than for married women (Stack, 1998). Several studies have shown that being married provides more advantages in terms of psychological and physiological well-being for men than for women (Ross and Mirovsky, 1990). The findings that men have greater health benefits from marriage mainly rely on three large prospective studies which initially assessed men's and women's marital and health status and then followed them for many years. In all three studies, unmarried men had a greater mortality risk than married men over the 9 to 15 years they were followed (Berkman and Syme, 1979; House et al., 1982; Shye et al., 1995, see Helgeson, 2005). In contrast, marital status did not predict mortality among women in any of these studies. Yet, it is not clear whether the findings of associations between partnership and mortality are also transferable to outcomes such as subjective quality of life. One explanation for the association between partner status and health status is provided by social support. Social support as a buffer after stressful life events has been described repeatedly in stress research and has a long tradition in health psychology (Rieckmann, 2003). Married men and women report higher levels of social support than unmarried individuals (Ross, 1995). As the support through marriage is greater for men, marriage may confer a greater health benefit for men than for women (Stroebe and Stroebe, 1983). This is particularly true for emotional support. Men are more likely to name their spouses as their primary confidants and receive more emotional support from their spouse than vice versa women from their husbands (Tower and Kasl, 1996). Another reason for the poorer well-being of individuals without a partner could have to do with the occurrence of stressful life events (Ensel, 1986). Events such as divorce, separation or the death of a partner are normally experienced as extremely stressful and entail stress in the long term. When life events and social support are controlled for in the analyses, the differences between married and unmarried people vanish. Partnership seems to have protective effects whereas the loss of a partner has negative effects. How these effects are moderated by gender and age so far remains unclear, but there is some evidence that the protective effects are stronger in men than in women (Siegel and Kuykendall, 1990).

**Death of a Spouse**

With growing age, people increasingly have to deal with losses. Usually, women are confronted with adverse life events such as death of the spouse earlier than men. If marriage provides protective effects it may be assumed that the loss of a spouse leads to negative effects. These negative effects may result from the loss of resources due to the death of the spouse (Helgeson, 2005). To interpret these effects is not simple because the majority of studies are cross-sectional. In a review conducted by Stroebe & Stroebe (1983), men whose spouse had died either had higher depression levels than women in the comparable situation or no differences were found. This result differs from epidemiological studies, which always report higher depression levels in women. The authors hence conclude that widowerhood leads to higher levels of distress in men than widowhood in women. Similar results have been reported concerning physical and mental health. Widowed persons were less healthy than married persons – the differences being more marked in men than in women. This difference in stress experience became even more pronounced over time. Van Groothest et al. (1999) demonstrated that the gender difference in recently widowed people was relatively small but increased over the years. Likewise, in a study by Lee et al. (1998) men and women differed in depression levels only 3 years after being widowed. This may indicate that women recover more easily from widowhood. One explanation could be that women have greater social networks, whose importance increases with growing age. With the death of their spouse men often lose their only source of emotional support. Women, too, may have more support because for them asking for support is generally accepted. Generally in marriage it is the woman who cultivates the social contacts of the couple. Therefore, for men the social network as an important source of support is likely to decrease with widowerhood. In contrast, marriage for women is also linked to "costs" with women often providing more support than they receive. This may be another explanation for the finding that women experience less stress than men after being widowed.

**Domestic Work**

There is some evidence that recovery after CABG operation proceeds differently in male and female patients. For example, the probability of women taking part in rehabilitation activities is lower than for men. Differences in personal circumstances appear to influence the reasons reported by men and women for not participating in outpatient rehabilitation programmes, such as in supervised exercise groups. Men and women differ in the reasons given. The main reasons for non-participation cited by men include a lack of interest. Women most often give practical reasons for non-participation, stating for example that the programme is too far from their home, that they have to take care of relatives or that they have no means of transportation (Härtel, 2003; Ades et al., 1992).

Normally a gender-specific division of work remains after the diagnosis of CHD or an operation. Wilke et al. (1995) postulate that patients diagnosed with CHD are generally able to perform normal household tasks without exposing themselves to the risk of complications. In this study, however, the cardiac event already dated back 2-11 years. At this time most patients are indeed able to attend to their habitual activities. However, often the resumption of household activities reported by women does not correspond to the level of functioning at that time (King, 2000). Therefore it may happen that, because of their caring for relatives or doing the domestic work, women overlook physical warning signals. Possibly premature resumption of habitual activities has an impact on the long-term recovery (Rose et al., 1996). Do women overextend themselves in the early phase after discharge from hospital, when they are at the highest risk of complications? Only few studies have analyzed the association between household activities shortly after a cardiac event. Rose et al. (1996) conducted a prospective cross-sectional study (15 men, 15 women) and stated that partners of female patients increased their time spent on household activities in the first weeks after the MI of their spouse. But already 10 weeks after the MI female patients assumed significantly more household tasks than their partners. The support provided by the partners was restricted to the time span directly after the discharge from hospital. In contrast, male patients experienced a significant release from household duties after the MI, which allowed them a longer recovery period after the cardiac event. Generally it seemed difficult for patients to relinquish traditional roles that conform to gender stereotypes. Lemos et al. (2003) assessed cardiovascular symptoms and activities resumed, using a longitudinal design. The relationship between symptoms and activities differed markedly between men and women. In men, the associations were negative: the more symptoms they reported, the more they reduced their activities. In women, the reported symptoms seemed to be independent of their activities. The authors therefore concluded that women generally attended less to their symptoms and needs. This behaviour pattern might place women at special risk, since domestic work tends to be performed consecutively, being concentrated on a certain period, rather than being evenly distributed across the day. In the early phase of recovery, when patients are instructed to avoid exertion of the upper part of the body, this behaviour pattern could represent an increased risk (Lemos et al., 2003). In Germany, so far, there is little research examining the relationship between stress due to household activities and MI or bypass surgery.

Even though gender differences concerning anxiety, depression and social support are well-known in the psychological literature, the vast majority of studies done on psychological factors in CABG have not investigated these differences or have not reported gender-specific results. Generally, women display more anxiety and more depressive symptoms before surgery. Studies on gender differences in recovery with respect to depression and anxiety have yielded conflicting results. Moreover, the relationship between an early resumption of housework, social support and recovery is not yet fully understood. The independent influence of depression on cardiac events has been the object of numerous studies. So far there are three main limitations of existing research in this area: (1) the majority of studies have not addressed depression or quality of life among *women* with cardiac disease; (2) the studies have been primarily cross-sectional; (3) some studies did not utilize standard indicators of health-related quality of life, making the results difficult to compare.

In this context, two gender differences are particularly interesting: on one hand, women exhibit higher depression rates throughout the population; on the other hand, they seem more vulnerable towards the adverse effects of depression on the cardiovascular system. Additionally they have, on average, more clinical risk factors and report less social support, both factors being associated with depression. Being married seems to provide more advantages for men, while, accordingly, being widowed makes men more vulnerable.

## 1.3 Outcome Measures

In this section, both clinical and psychosocial outcome parameters are discussed.

### 1.3.1 Mortality

In the present study, mortality was used as the objective outcome parameter. The majority of studies reported higher mortality rates in women compared to men. Gender differences in mortality have been outlined in detail in section 1.2.

### 1.3.2 Quality of Life

In recent years, in addition to the objective measures of cardiovascular status, health-related quality of life has gained increasing attention as a psychosocial outcome parameter in studies of cardiovascular disease. Meanwhile, guidelines published by the American College of Cardiology and the American Heart Association suggest that, if the decision for bypass surgery is to be made, not only mortality rates shall be focussed on. Rather it becomes more and more important to turn one's attention to the improvement of the quality of life (Eagle and Guyton, 1999). There is no general opinion about what quality of life means or how it can be measured. Most researchers agree that quality of life is a multidimensional construct, but as yet there is no agreement about which dimensions should be assessed. Major domains with regard to health-related quality of life assessment are subjectively perceived physical functioning, emotional status, social functioning and general perceptions of health and well-being. Thus, health-related quality of life is a reflection of the patients' perception and reaction to their health status and social aspects of their lives (Duits et al., 1997). One main goal of CABG is to improve oxygen supply and thereby to improve physical activity. This, in turn, has consequences for work, leisure, social activities and mood. Successful surgery enables most patients to resume a much fuller way of everyday life (King et al., 1993, Allen et al., 1990, Mayou and Bryant, 1987). How the subjective quality of life is improved by surgery has been shown in several studies (for a review see Duits et al., 1997). For some patients, however, outcome for quality of life can be disappointing despite successful surgery (Langeluddecke et al., 1989). Age, education, comorbidity and – less consistently – gender have been shown to predict quality of life. For example, Bute at al. (2003) showed that women already before surgery had greater psychosocial and physical constraints than men. Though the quality of life improved within the whole sample over the following time period, female patients showed a significantly poorer outcome than male patients at 1-year follow-up in several key areas of quality of life. After adjustment for baseline differences a significant gender difference remained. This means that preoperative differences only contribute in part to the postoperatively observed differences. The findings of Bute et al. are contrary to the findings of Hunt et al. (2000) who could not find any significant gender differences on either subscale of the SF-36. However, this sample was much smaller than that of Bute et al. and did not include baseline data. King (2000) in her study concluded that gender did not play a consistent role as a predictor of biopsychological recovery. Women recovered as well as men from bypass surgery. Finally, Sjoland et al. (1999) reported a lower level of quality of life in women but no gender-dependent differences in *changes* of quality of life over time. In this study, except for age, preoperatively existing differences were not controlled for.

In recent years, there has been a proliferation of interest in long-term psychological adaptation and in different aspects of quality of life after CABG. Even so there is still a lack of prospective research studying certain aspects of life such as mental state or social functioning. So far, little attention has been given to the way in which the various dimensions of quality of life might affect one another. Such knowledge could provide more insight into the concept and its clinical relevance. As yet, only few studies have focused on gender differences in outcome after CABG.

These studies have yielded conflicting results with respect to gender, which may be partly due to different instruments and different sample sizes.

### 1.3.3 Depression

In section 1.3.2 the role of depression as a risk factor was described. However, patients also may react to stress and adverse health conditions with depressive symptoms. Thus depression may be a risk factor and an outcome parameter at the same time. An operation, for example, is a stressor, which often interacts with depression and anxiety. Analyzing depression in connection with CABG poses three distinct problems. First, depression is a prevalent condition in the normal population, the lifetime prevalence ranging from 5.2 to 17.1% (Weissman et al., 1996). This great range is due to different methods applied to the assessment of depression, different criteria of diagnosis and differing knowledge of interviewers. In addition to these differences the prevalence in women is about twice as high as in men. It is more frequent in people with a lower socioeconomic status and in young adults (Davison & Neale, 2002). The second problem is that patients undergoing CABG often have a clinical history of depression that has persisted for many years. Symptoms such as fatigue, dyspnea or general exhaustion may cause and interact with depressive symptoms. The third problem is the operation itself. In addition to the baseline condition the cardiac operation may be experienced as a life-threatening procedure (Bresser et al., 1993). Some patients fail to adapt to this procedure and increased anxiety and depression have been noted postoperatively (Langeluddecke et al., 1989).

McKhann et al. (1997) reported that 50% of the patients who were depressive prior to the surgery were still depressive after surgery. In contrast, only 13% of the non-depressive patients were depressive 1 month after surgery, the number decreasing to 9% 1 year after surgery.

Given the high rate of depression in epidemiological studies, the relationship between gender and adverse outcomes after CABG surgery may be population-rooted. However, the predictive direction is not always unambiguous. Depression may be a predictor that directly and indirectly triggers adverse outcomes. Depression may also be seen as an outcome parameter. As such, it may be a reaction to a poor health status or to the operation.

Women preoperatively display a poorer quality of life. However, the question of whether women do worse postoperatively in terms of quality of life has yielded conflicting results. As an outcome parameter, depression may be a reaction to a poor physical health status. Stress related to surgery may also lead to an increase in depressive symptoms. However, the predictive relationship between physical functioning and depression is yet unclear.

# 2 HYPOTHESES

Here, the central research questions and hypotheses are summarized. The main objective of the study was to evaluate risk factors for health-related quality of life and mortality after CABG in men and women. The empirical and theoretical considerations that underlie the hypotheses were outlined in detail in chapter 1.

The research questions are divided into three groups. The first group concerns the general question of how risk factors, quality of life and mortality rates differ between men and women and which relationships are expected. Assumptions about levels and changes of outcome variables are formulated. The second group deals with hypotheses concerning the moderator status of gender. Finally, the third group relates to the mediator status of risk factors.

## 2.1 Gender Differences in Risk Factors and Outcomes

Previous studies have shown a variety of gender differences with respect to risk factors and outcomes, from which the following hypotheses are derived:

1. Women differ from men in their sociodemographic profile and have a poorer physical health status both before and after surgery. They also differ from men in their mental health status (higher depression and anxiety scores).

2. After surgery, the average quality of life and depression compared to the conditions before surgery improves in both men and women. Improvement in these factors over time is less marked in women than in men.

3. Women have a higher all-cause mortality rate in the first year after CABG surgery.

4. In both genders, psychosocial, clinical and sociodemographic risk factors are associated with both mortality and physical functioning.

5. After CABG women return to housework prematurely and thereby impair their recovery.

6. Preoperative depression influences postoperative physical functioning and vice versa.

## 2.2 Moderator Hypotheses

Several studies have demonstrated that risk factors have a stronger impact on wellbeing in women than in men. This leads to the following "moderator hypotheses" (for an explanation of the rationale see section 4.1.2).

1. Depression, clinical risk factors (diabetes, high cholesterol levels, smoking, and hypertension) and sociodemographic factors (low education level) are more strongly associated with mortality and lower physical functioning in women than in men.

2. Living without a partner is more strongly associated with mortality and a lower physical functioning in men than in women.

## 2.3 Mediator Hypotheses

In addition to *stronger* associations between risk factors and outcomes (see section 2.2 above), women are expected to be more often depressive, have lower levels of education, are older and have a less favourable risk profile. This higher prevalence of risk factors in women is expected to contribute to an explanation of the gender gap in mortality and physical functioning. This leads to the following compound "mediator hypothesis" (for an explanation of the rationale see section 4.1.2).

3. Depression, age, education level, partner status and clinical risk factors mediate the relationship between gender and mortality as well as between gender and physical functioning.

# 3 METHOD

In this chapter, methodological details are presented. First, the recruitment of participants and the procedure of data collection are described. Second, an overview of the demographic, medical and psychosocial measurements is given. Subsequently, a description of the sample with a focus on the drop-out is given. Finally, the main statistical procedures are discussed.

The study was part of a larger prospective study carried out by the Competence Network of Heart Failure (Kompetenznetz Herzinsuffizienz) funded by the German Federal Ministry of Education and Research (BMBF).

## 3.1 Participants

Here, details of the recruitment procedure are given, followed by inclusion and exclusion criteria of the present study.

### 3.1.1 Recruitment Procedures

After approval by the Charité – Universitätsmedizin Berlin (Medical University of Berlin) Ethics Board was granted, recruitment of participants for the study took place at the Deutsches Herzzentrum Berlin, Department of Cardiothoracic and Vascular Surgery. Potential candidates were identified through daily screening of the admission records and were given information about the purpose of the study. Anonymity was assured. If a patient was interested in participating, he or she was asked to sign forms for participation. The questionnaire itself was given to the patients at latest 1 day before surgery with a short explanation of how to complete it. Clinical data such as laboratory values or course of surgery were derived from the medical records and case report forms and were documented by the study investigators. Two months and 1 year after surgery, respectively, eligible and consenting patients were sent another questionnaire. At any time the patients could withdraw their consent and drop out of the study without giving reasons.

### 3.1.2 Inclusion/Exclusion Criteria

Patients with coronary heart disease (CHD), with or without signs of heart failure, undergoing bypass surgery were included in the study. Other inclusion criteria were a minimum age of 18 years and written consent to participation. Exclusion criteria pertained to a lacking ability to read or answer the study questionnaires (e.g. dementia, difficulties with the language). If a patient was excluded for these or other reasons, age, sex and reason for exclusion were documented.

## 3.2 Measurements

For the present study, the questionnaire was developed according to theoretical principles on the basis of validated instruments. It contained sociodemographic, clinical and psychosocial variables. Sociodemographic data and a number of clinical variables were assessed once prior to surgery. Shortly after surgery additional medical data were gathered from surgery records. Anxiety, depression, quality of life and social support were assessed at all three time points surrounding surgery. Household chores were measured once 2 months after surgery. Table 2 exemplifies the study design.

**Table 2. Study Design**

| Variables | T1 (1 day before surgery) | T2 (2 months after surgery) | T3 (1 year after surgery) |
|---|---|---|---|
| Sociodemographic data | X | | |
| Clinical parameters | X | | |
| Anxiety and depression | X | X | X |
| Quality of life | X | X | X |
| Housework | | X | |
| Social support | X | X | X |

### 3.2.1 Outcome Parameters

All-cause (not cardiovascular) 1-year mortality was selected as an objective outcome variable. Subjective end-points included the physical functioning subscale from the SF-36 health status survey and depression from the patient health questionnaire (PHQ) (for detailed descriptions see 3.2.4).

### 3.2.2 Sociodemographic Data

A series of sociodemographic variables was assessed before surgery: date of birth, gender, family status and education level. The final coding followed the guidelines of the Working Group on Epidemiological Studies (Ahrens et al., 1998). Therein family status was treated as a dichotomous variable: living with a partner versus no partner (single, divorced, widowed, separated). A three-level categorical variable was created to indicate the different levels of (vocational) education: (1) No vocational training (2) Apprenticeship (3) Academic. Vocational education in this context was used as an indicator for socio-economic status (SES).

### 3.2.3 Clinical Data

Several clinical variables indicated the objective health status of participants. Clinical risk factors were collected prospectively at preoperative admission and included cardiovascular risk factors, prior cardiac interventions, operative status and coexisting illnesses. Intraoperative data (e.g. bypass time, intraoperative complications) and postoperative data (e.g. postoperative infarction, duration of intensive care unit stay) were derived from the medical records. In order to maintain as much information as possible from the medical dataset, but nevertheless to reduce the total number of risk factors, the EuroSCORE (Cardiac Operative Risk Evaluation) was calculated according to the STS Risk Stratification Analysis Algorithm (Nashef et al., 1999). The additive EuroSCORE model has been shown to work well across many European countries and has become a widely accepted and well-validated instrument over the past few years (Roques et al., 2000). The EuroSCORE focuses on perioperative risk factors to predict the risk of mortality after heart surgery. The Framingham Score was developed to predict the risk of developing coronary heart disease or myocardial infarction. This was not the goal of this study. However, as the Framingham Score summarizes clinical risk factors for heart disease such as cholesterol, hypertension, smoking and diabetes and is accepted as a well-validated instrument (Wilson et al., 1998) it was used in order to reduce the total number of these risk factors.

### 3.2.4 Psychosocial Variables

Psychosocial factors were assigned by means of self-report questionnaires, including the Patient Health Questionnaire PHQ, Hospital Anxiety and Depression Scale HADS-D, Quality of Life SF-36, "Social Support" from the Enhancing Recovery in Heart Patients ENRICHD, and the Household Questionnaire. The internal consistency was calculated using Cronbach's α. Table 4 at the end of this chapter displays the psychometric properties (Cronbach's α, skewness, kurtosis) for each scale.

### Anxiety

The Hospital Anxiety and Depression scale (HADS) (Zigmond and Snaith, 1983; German version Herrmann et al., 1995) was used to assess anxiety at all 3 measurement points. The subscale anxiety is specifically designed as a screening instrument for physically ill patients and does not include somatic symptoms for the assessment of anxiety. It consists of seven items, with anxiety scores ranging from 0 to 21, higher scores indicating higher anxiety. Scores over 8 indicate that patients are likely to experience an anxiety level of clinical relevance. Internal consistency ranged from $\alpha = 0.77$ to $\alpha = 0.84$ and was thus acceptable.

**Depression**

The Patient Health Questionnaire (PHQ) (Spitzer et al., 1999; German version: Löwe et al., 2002) was used to assess depression. The depression items that form the nine-item depression module "PHQ-9" directly display diagnostic criteria from the DSM-IV for major depression. The German version has shown excellent reliability and validity (Löwe et al., 2004). Items are endorsed on a 4-point scale with the response options "not at all", "several days", "more than half the days", and "nearly every day". The score ranges from 0 to 27, with higher scores indicating a higher level of depression. Major depression is diagnosed when at least 5 symptoms of depression occur at more than half the days including at least one of the two main diagnostic symptoms for major depressive disorder ("little interest or pleasure in doing things", or "feeling down, depressed or hopeless"). Since distinguishing between clinically relevant versus non-relevant cases was not the explicit goal of this study, the PHQ score was used in the continuous form in order to maintain the full information. As the scales were non-normally distributed, a square-root transformation was fitted to the data to obtain an optimal solution. Internal consistencies of the PHQ-9 ranged from Cronbach's $\alpha = 0.81$ to $\alpha = 0.92$ and were thus within an acceptable range.

**Social Support**

Social support was assessed by participant's scores on the Enhancing Recovery in Coronary Heart Disease (ENRICHD) Social Support Instrument (ESSI). The ESSI is a six-item self-report measure used in the ENRICHD trial (Berkman et al., 1992). It has been used in recent clinical trials and has shown acceptable internal consistency and validity. Five items measuring emotional social support were selected from the original scale and translated to German by the author of this study (Table 3). One item, which assessed instrumental support rather than emotional support, was excluded from the scale. The translation process included a forward and backward translation. The 5 emotional social support items and the German translation are presented in Table 3. The scale was tested within a pilot study (N = 50), which was conducted at the "Deutsches Herzzentrum Berlin" (German Heart Institute). The results showed an acceptable reliability (Cronbach's $\alpha = 0.89$) and indicated that all patients understood the items properly.

Items are endorsed on a 5-point scale with the response options ranging from "for none of the time" to "for all of the time". The score ranges from 5 to 25, with higher scores indicating greater social support. As the social support scales were non-normally distributed, a square-root transformation was fitted to the data to obtain an optimal solution. Internal consistencies ranged from Cronbach's $\alpha = 0.90$ to $\alpha = 0.93$ and were thus satisfying (Table 4).

**Table 3. Original Wording of the ESSI and German Translation**

| Item | Original Scale | German Translation |
|------|----------------|--------------------|
| ESSI 1 | Is there someone available to you who you can count on to listen when you need to talk? | Wenn Sie ein Gespräch brauchen, gibt es jemanden, der Ihnen richtig zuhört? |
| ESSI 2 | Is there someone available to give you good advice about a problem? | Gibt es jemanden, der Ihnen einen guten Rat gibt, wenn sie ein Problem haben? |
| ESSI 3 | Is there someone available to you who shows you love and affection? | Gibt es jemanden, der Ihnen Liebe und Zuneigung zeigt? |
| ESSI 5 | Can you count on anyone to provide you with emotional support, such as talking over problems or helping you make difficult decisions? | Können Sie auf jemanden zählen, der Sie emotional unterstützt (z.B. mit Ihnen über Ihre Sorgen spricht oder Ihnen bei schwierigen Entscheidungen hilft)? |
| ESSI 6 | Do you have as much contact as you would like with someone you feel close to, someone you can trust and confide in? | Haben Sie zu einem Menschen, dem Sie sich nahe fühlen und dem Sie vertrauen, soviel Kontakt, wie Sie sich das wünschen? |

**Domestic Work**

The self-report measure of household stress and time spent on household tasks was adapted from a recently developed instrument: the Housework and Family Activity Scale" (Worringen et al., 2001). Patients were asked using single items whether they performed household activities, how much time they spent on these activities, how much stress they experienced by their housework and whether they could count on support from anyone for these activities. The patients were informed that the term "housework" included shopping, cooking, cleaning, washing, gardening and car maintenance. The following single items were included in the present study (German version in parentheses):

- Do you perform housework in your own household?

  [Erledigen Sie in Ihrem Haushalt Hausarbeiten?]

  (response options: no/yes)

- How many hours do you generally need for the housework?

  [Wieviel Zeit benötigen Sie für die Arbeit im eigenen Haushalt im Normalfall?]

  (response options: more than 6 hours daily/3 to 6 hours daily/1 to 3 hours daily/less than one hour daily)

- Who supports you with the housework?

  [Wer unterstützt Sie bei der Haushaltsarbeit?]

  (response options: my partner/my parents/my children/others/nobody)

- How demanding is the housework for you?

  [Wie stark fühlen Sie sich durch die Haushaltsarbeit beansprucht?]

  (response options: 4-point scale ranging from "not at all" to "much")

**Quality of Life**

In order to include a subjective measure of the health status, the subscale "physical functioning" from the 36-item Medical Outcomes Study Short-Form health survey (SF-36) was used at all three measurement points. The SF-36 was developed and authorized by Ware et al. (1993). Excellent psychometric properties (reliability, validity and sensitivity) have been reported for the SF-36 (Ware, 1993). The German version (Bullinger and Kirchberger, 1998) has been tested with numerous patients in Germany. The subscale "physical functioning" consists of ten items eliciting concrete responses about physical limitations due to health, such as using stairs, lifting and carrying groceries. The format of response choices for the subscale "physical functioning" varies from "yes, strongly restricted" to "no, not restricted at all". Raw scores of the subscale were transformed to a score ranging from 0 (severe impairment) to 100 (no impairment).

**Table 4. Overview over Psychometric Properties**

| | Number of Items | Full Sample N= 579 | | | Continuer Sample N= 355 | | |
|---|---|---|---|---|---|---|---|
| | | Cronbach's $\alpha$ | Skewness | Kurtosis | Cronbach's $\alpha$ | Skewness | Kurtosis |
| PF T1 | 10 | 0.92 | 0.00 | -0.99 | 0.91 | -0.11 | -0.96 |
| PF T2 | 10 | | | | 0.91 | -0.50 | 0.53 |
| PF T3 | 10 | | | | 0.93 | -0.66 | -0.70 |
| Depression T1 | 9 | 0.82 | 1.12 (-0.06)[1] | 1.23 (0.05)[1] | 0.81 | 1.10 (0.67)[1] | 0.99 (-0.45)[1] |
| Depression T2 | 9 | | | | 0.92 | 1.48 (0.99)[1] | 2.69 (0.13)[1] |
| Depression T3 | 9 | | | | 0.86 | 1.54 (0.91)[1] | 2.68 (-0.12)[1] |
| Anxiety T1 | 7 | 0.77 | 0.55 | -0.29 | 0.77 | 0.52 | -0.26 |
| Anxiety T2 | 7 | | | | 0.84 | 1.02 | 0.95 |
| Anxiety T3 | 7 | | | | 0.84 | 1.05 | 0.75 |
| Social Support T1 | 5 | 0.90 | -1.42 (-0.04)[1] | 1.65 (0.34)[1] | 0.90 | -1.37 (-0.03)[1] | 1.46 (0.26)[1] |
| Social Support T2 | 5 | | | | 0.91 | -1.74 (0.07)[1] | 2.72 (0.26)[1] |
| Social Support T3 | 5 | | | | 0.93 | -1.62 (0.18)[1] | 2.28 (0.01)[1] |

Note. (1) Numbers in brackets show skewness and kurtosis after square root transformation
PF Physical Functioning

## 3.3 General Statistical Procedures

This section details the treatment of missing data and the main statistical methods used in the present study. Statistical analyses were performed using SPSS 14.00 for Windows, AMOS 5.0 (Arbuckle, 1999) and NORM (Schafer, 1999). All tests for statistical significance were two-sided: those with an alpha level of at least $p \leq 0.05$ were considered statistically significant; an alpha level of $p \leq 0.10$ and $\geq 0.05$ was considered marginal.

### 3.3.1 Missing Values

Missing data in psychosomatic medicine are omnipresent, but still pose an often underestimated problem. One can distinguish unit non-response, which occurs when the entire data collection fails (for example if a person refuses to participate), from item non-response, which means that the person partially answered the questionnaire but did not respond to certain individual items (Tabachnick and Fidell, 2007).

In this study, in order to avoid a reduction of the sample, the exclusion of incomplete variables (listwise or pairwise deletion) was rejected (see Barnes et al., 2006). With regard to the underlying assumptions as well as the amount and pattern of the data, a procedure that performs maximum-likelihood estimation on the matrix of incomplete data using the Expectation Maximization (EM) algorithm was chosen. All missing data analyses and the imputation of missing data were conducted using the software NORM (Schafer, 1999). Roughly 10% of the cases had missing values on psychosocial variables. On each variable, approximately 2-7% of the values were missing. The matrix of missingness provided by NORM did not reveal a concentration of missing values in any critical subset of the data within the respective waves, the missing values being well spread amongst variables and cases. After examination of the data summary, missing data were estimated on item level by the EM procedure, using all remaining items of the respective scale as predictors. Data were only replaced within one wave of data collection. The EM algorithm is a general technique for fitting models to incomplete data based on a process with two steps: (1) the Expectation (E) step in which missing statistics are replaced by their expected values given the observed data, using estimated values for the parameters; and (2) the Maximization (M) step where the parameters are updated by their maximum-likelihood estimates, given the statistics obtained from the E-step. The procedure is run iteratively until convergence is obtained.

### 3.3.2 Statistical Procedures

In a first step bivariate associations were tested by Pearson's correlations, t-tests for independent and dependent samples and, if non-parametric, with $\chi^2$-tests. To allow for an examination of longitudinal data, multiple regression, repeated-measures analyses of variance, and structural equation modelling were performed.

All distributions were screened for normality, skewness and kurtosis. If variables were not normally distributed and if the shape of the distribution was not satisfying, transformation of variables was performed according to Tabachnick and Fidell (2007). In most cases of non-normally distributed variables, the optimal solution was obtained by performing a square root transformation. If departure from normality was severe and no transformation led to a satisfying result, the variable was dichotomized.

## Multiple Regression

In order to assess the relationship between one dependent variable and several independent variables, regression analyses were used. Logistic regression was performed to predict a discrete outcome, linear multiple regression when the outcome variable was continuous. Depending on the research question, regression analyses were performed either hierarchically (if the inclusion of control variables was intended) or by backward selection (if the identification of main predictors was intended). If changes between measurement points were the objects of interest, the value of the outcome variable at the first measurement point was entered in the first step, thus producing a residual change value. Interactions were tested by entering the two single predictors in the first step and the interaction term in the next step. To avoid problems with multicollinearity in regression analyses with interaction terms, the respective components of each interaction term were, in accordance with Aiken and West (1991), centred around the sample mean and then, in order to build the interaction term, multiplied. According to Baron and Kenny (1986), regression analyses were also used to test hypotheses that are concerned with possible mediation. The detailed rationale behind moderation and mediation is worked out in section 4.1.2.

## Repeated Measures Analyses

A multivariate approach to repeated-measures ANOVA was used to test hypotheses about differences between two or more means concerning different measurement points and gender. Generally, gender was used as the between-subject variable or the independent variable respectively, while repeated measures of the outcome variable were treated as dependent variables. Thereby, ANOVA provides tests of groups, trials and their interaction. Bonferroni adjustment was chosen for adjustment of alpha-levels when post-hoc tests were performed. Because sample sizes for the main between-subjects variable, i.e. gender, were unequal, special attention was paid to the homogeneity of variances. If Levine's test for homogeneity indicated unequal variances, Tamhane's test was applied for post-hoc comparisons between groups. If the assumption of sphericity was not met in repeated measures analyses, degrees of freedom were adjusted within the F-test by performing the Greenhouse-Geisser correction.

## Structural Equation Modelling

Cross-sectional and prospective relationships between depression and physical functioning were tested in a cross-lagged panel design using structural equation modelling (SEM). There are two main advantages of SEM. First, SEM is able to estimate all parameters simultaneously and can provide an overall test of model fit. Second, SEM allows for adjustment of measurement error, which requires specification of a measurement model that includes latent (theoretical constructs) and observed variables (measured variables). In order to use this utility, variables were understood as latent constructs in this process. At all measurement points, the latent constructs were estimated by two randomly selected split-half "subtests" (Arbuckle and Wottke, 1995).

## 3.4 Sample

This section provides information on sample size and attrition rates. Possible effects of attrition were explored by using $\chi^2$-tests or t-tests, respectively. These analyses are followed by a description of both the full sample and the continuer sample (patients who took part at all measurement points).

### 3.4.1 Sample Size

The full sample of the present study at T1 comprised 579 patients (21.1% women). 155 (26.8%) of these 579 participants failed to provide data at measurement point T2 and another 69 (11.9%) participants at measurement point T3. If participants did not contribute to the second measurement point, they were nevertheless contacted at measurement point T3. Three hundred and fifty-five patients answered questionnaires at *all* three measurement occasions, which corresponds to 61.3% of the full sample (see Figure 1).

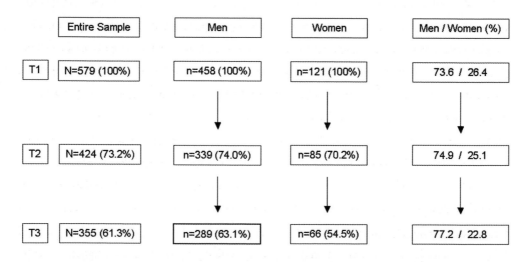

*Figure 1. Participation Rates*

A total of 224 patients were excluded from the longitudinal analyses in the present study because they did not contribute to either the second or the third wave of data collection. Table 5 shows the drop-out reasons for men and women separately. For 13.9% of these patients no information about the drop-out was obtainable; 6.6% of the patients died during the first year after surgery, for 6.7% of the patients important parts of the questionnaires were missing, 4.3% withdrew their consent to participate and another 7.6% completed the questionnaires for the third time point, but failed to send the questionnaires at the second time point. Within this setting it seems likely that the factors that prevented participants from sending the questionnaires were confounded systematically with the major outcome variables in the present study. Therefore, the decision was made to replace missing data within the same waves rather than replacing missing values over different waves of the data collection (see section 4.4.1).

**Table 5. Reasons for Drop-out**

|  | Entire Sample N= 589 | % | Male n= 458 | % | Female n= 121 | % |
|---|---|---|---|---|---|---|
| Unable to be contacted | 79 | 13.9 | 63 | 13.7 | 16 | 13.2 |
| Died during follow-up | 39 | 6.6 | 24 | 5.2 | 15 | 12.4 |
| Questionnaire not complete or received late | 38 | 6.7 | 28 | 6.3 | 10 | 8.3 |
| Withdrawal of consent due to poor health condition | 25 | 4.3 | 18 | 3.9 | 7 | 5.8 |
| T2 questionnaire missing | 44 | 7.6 | 37 | 8.1 | 7 | 5.8 |
| Total | 224 | 38.7 | 170 | 36.8 | 55 | 45.5 |

### 3.4.2 Drop-out Analysis

In order to gain insight into potential effects of attrition, selected sample characteristics – physical functioning, depression, anxiety, partner status, age and LVEF – for all participants at T1 as well as for continuers and non-continuers are shown in Table 6. The drop-out-analyses were calculated for men and women separately. Differences between the groups were calculated by t-tests for continuous data and $\chi^2$-square for categorical data.

The continuer sample did not differ from the non-continuer sample with respect to age. However, continuers were to a higher proportion living with a partner, had a better LVEF, a better physical functioning and lower anxiety and depression scores. In addition to an examination of the full sample, the effects of continuation were examined for men and women separately. Within the male sample, continuers also had a better LVEF, a better physical functioning and fewer symptoms of anxiety and depression. In accordance with the full sample, those men, who took part at all measurement points were more often living with a partner.

Within the female sample, the same pattern emerged. Continuing women showed a better LVEF, a better physical functioning and were less depressive, whereas the differences in anxiety and partner status did not reach significance. However, comparing the full sample with the continuer sample, the differences between men and women were less marked on all variables except for the LVEF. This means, that the danger of an α-error (exaggerating differences between the two genders due to drop-out) is limited.

**Table 6. Distributions for the Full Sample, Continuers and Non-Continuers**

| Characteristic | Full Sample T1 N= 579 | Continuers n= 224 | Non-Continuers n= 355 | $\chi^2/t$ | df | p |
|---|---|---|---|---|---|---|
| **Entire Sample** | | | | | | |
| Age | 66.33±9.01 | 66.26±8.29 | 66.46±10.07 | -0.24 | 577 | n.s. |
| With Partner (%) | 72.4 | 77.2 | 64.7 | 10.64 | 1 | ** |
| LVEF | 53.63±14.5 | 55.28±14.6 | 50.95±14.4 | 3.49 | 577 | ** |
| Physical functioning | 51.37±26.7 | 54.32±25.9 | 46.66±27.5 | -3.38 | 577 | ** |
| depression | 6.43±4.8 | 5.77±4.29 | 7.47±5.33 | 4.21 | 577 | ** |
| anxiety | 5.92±3.8 | 5.55±4.0 | 6.51±3.7 | -2.94 | 577 | ** |
| **Male sample** | | | | | | |
| Age | 65.26±8.6 | 65.62 ± 7.89 | 64.64 ± 9.80 | 0.99 | 456 | n.s. |
| With Partner (%) | 81.0 | 84.8 | 74.6 | 7.24 | 1 | ** |
| LVEF | 53.75±14.5 | 54.8±14.1 | 51.7±14.9 | 1.40 | 456 | * |
| Physical functioning | 54.16±26.4 | 56.01±26.0 | 50.90±26.84 | -2.02 | 456 | * |
| Depression | 5.97±4.5 | 5.51±4.1 | 6.8±5.1 | 2.83 | 456 | ** |
| Anxiety | 5.63±3.8 | 5.34±3.9 | 6.13±3.6 | -2.17 | 456 | * |
| **Female sample** | | | | | | |
| Age | 70.4±9.3 | 69.06 ± 9.5 | 72.02 ± 8.9 | -1.75 | 118 | n.s. |
| With Partner (%) | 39.7 | 43.9 | 34.5 | 1.10 | 1 | n.s. |
| LVEF | 53.17±14.5 | 57.01 | 48.55 | 2.59 | 118 | ** |
| Physical functioning | 40.83±25.6 | 46.74±24.4 | 33.73±25.4 | -0.86 | 119 | ** |
| Depression | 8.17±5.4 | 6.91±4.8 | 9.69±5.5 | 2.93 | 119 | ** |
| Anxiety | 7.02±3.9 | 6.44±4.0 | 7.72±3.7 | -1.80 | 118 | n.s. |

Notes. +p < 0.10 *p < 0.05 **p < 0.01 ***p < 0.001

### 3.4.3 Sociodemographic Data

The full sample comprised 458 men and 121 women (22%). In this sample, women were approximately 5 years older than men, with a slightly higher variance.

The vast majority of men (73.1%) were married compared to only 34.7% of women. In contrast only 7.2% of men were widowed, compared to 42.1% of women. More men than women (22.9% versus 14.9%) reported more than 12 years of school education which corresponds to the German "Fachhochschulreife" or "Abitur" and accordingly more men than women reported having university education (28.2% versus 17.4%).

**Table 7. Age and Sociodemographic Data of the Full Sample by Gender**

| Characteristic | Men n= 458 | Women n= 121 | $\chi^2/t$ | df | p |
|---|---|---|---|---|---|
| **Age** | | | -5.74 | 577 | *** |
| Mean | 65.26 | 70.40 | | | |
| SD | 8.63 | 9.30 | | | |
| Range | 36-85 | 40-92 | | | |
| **Marital status %** | | | | | |
| Married | 73.1 | 34.7 | 62.24 | 1 | *** |
| Single | 13.3 | 18.2 | 1.84 | 1 | n.s. |
| Divorced | 6.3 | 5.0 | 0.32 | 1 | n.s. |
| Widowed | 7.2 | 42.1 | 94.23 | 1 | *** |
| **Years of Education %** | | | | | |
| ≤9yrs (Hauptschule) | 53.1 | 62.8 | 3.68 | 1 | * |
| 10yrs (Realschule/Polytechnische Oberschule) | 24.0 | 22.3 | 0.15 | 1 | n.s. |
| ≥12yrs (Fachhochschulreife/Abitur) | 22.9 | 14.9 | 3.70 | 1 | * |
| **Qualification %** | | | | | |
| No vocational training | 4.6 | 25.6 | 51.81 | 1 | *** |
| Apprenticeship/trade school | 67.2 | 57.0 | 4.40 | 1 | * |
| College of higher education/university | 28.2 | 17.4 | 5.83 | 1 | * |

Notes. $+p < 0.10$ $*p < 0.05$ $**p < 0.01$ $***p < 0.001$

# 4 RESULTS

The goal of this thesis is to describe gender differences in coronary artery bypass graft (CABG) surgery associated with the outcome parameters *mortality*, *physical functioning* (as an indicator for subjective health-related quality of life) and *depression*. The description of results is divided into three main parts. In section 4.1, data from the full sample are analyzed with a focus on the outcome parameters physical functioning and mortality. In section 4.2, data of the continuer sample – the patients who contributed to all three measurement points – are analyzed, focusing on quality of life and depression. Finally, in section 4.3, the predictive relationship between physical functioning and depression is examined.

## 4.1 Predictors of Mortality and Physical Functioning Based on Preoperative Data

In this chapter, four stages of analysis are introduced to evaluate the extent to which the observed gender differences in physical functioning and mortality after bypass surgery are associated with pre-existing health characteristics, hospital complications and psychosocial risk factors. The first stage of analysis involves simple t-tests or $\chi^2$-tests used to compare the profiles and risk factors of male and female patients in the above three areas of interest. In addition, a comparison with the German norm sample of the SF 36 is provided. The second stage of analysis employs correlations and $\chi^2$-tests to determine associations between mortality and potential risk factors. The third stage explores possible interaction terms to assess whether risk factors are more closely related with mortality or physical functioning in either men or women. Finally, the fourth stage employs multiple logistic and multiple linear regression modelling to demonstrate the interplay of risk factors and their influence on physical functioning and mortality.

### 4.1.1 Description of Predictors

This section provides a comparison of the clinical and psychosocial profiles of men and women, using simple t-tests for continuous and $\chi^2$-tests for categorical data.

## Demographic and Social Factors

Women were, on average, 5 years older than men ($M_{men} = 65.26 \pm 8.63$; $M_{women} = 70.40 \pm 9.29$; t (577) = -5.74, p < 0.001). Fifty-eight percent of women were over 70 years old compared to 30% of men ($\chi^2 = 32.53$; p < 0.001). Women were more likely to live alone or to be widowed ($\chi^2 = 81.78$; p < 0.001) and had lower levels of education ($\chi^2 = 53.01$; p < 0.001). The structure of the analyzed data is depicted in Figure 2.

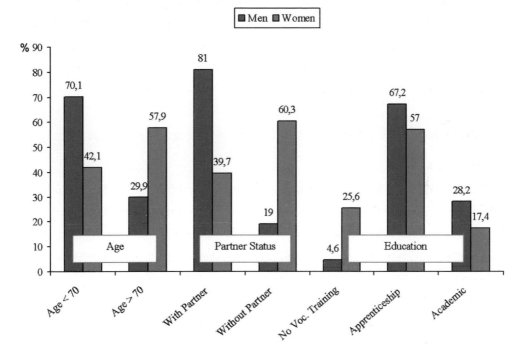

*Figure 2. Sociodemographic Characteristics by Gender: The Full Sample*

## Perioperative Health Status

Details of the baseline health status are presented in Table 8. The analysis yielded a significant gender difference with regard to congestive heart failure. A greater proportion of women suffered from congestive heart failure whereas differences in angina pectoris and left ventricular ejection fraction (LVEF) were not significant. More women than men were classified as having normal weight (BMI < 25). On average, men had a higher body mass index than women ($M_{men} = 27.64$ SD = 3,89, $M_{women} = 26.63$, SD = 4.52, t = 2.44, p < 0.01).

## Table 8. Gender Differences in Baseline Health Status: $\chi^2$-test

|  | Men n= 458 | Women n= 121 | $\chi^2$ | df | p |  |
|---|---|---|---|---|---|---|
| Angina pectoris % | 78.9 | 76.7 | 0.25 | 1 | 0.61 | n.s. |
| Congestive heart failure % | 29.3 | 38.7 | 3.87 | 1 | 0.05 | * |
| LVEF % |  |  |  |  |  |  |
| <30% | 7 | 6.6 | 0.01 | 1 | 0.95 | n.s. |
| 30-50% | 32.8 | 31.4 | 0.01 | 1 | 0.96 | n.s. |
| >50% | 60.3 | 62.0 | 0.01 | 1 | 0.97 | n.s. |
| BMI % |  |  |  |  |  |  |
| <25 kg/m$^2$ | 24.7 | 39.7 | 10.72 | 1 | 0.00 | *** |
| 25-29 kg/m$^2$ | 45.0 | 37.2 | 2.36 | 1 | 0.12 | n.s. |
| >30 kg/m$^2$ | 22.9 | 17.4 | 1.74 | 1 | 0.19 | n.s. |

Notes. n.s. non significant *p < 0.05 ***p < 0.001

LVEF: Left ventricular ejection fraction

BMI: Body mass index

## Clinical Risk Factors

As can be seen in Table 9, there were some gender differences in baseline risk factors. However, out of these risk factors only the gender difference in hypertension reached significance. Compared to women, more men stated that they had smoked or were still smoking. Women had more often undergone percutaneous coronary intervention (PCI), this difference being marginally significant.

## Table 9. Risk Factors of Coronary Heart Disease Compared by Gender: Significance of $\chi^2$-test

|  | Men n= 458 | Women n= 121 | $\chi^2$ | df | p |  |
|---|---|---|---|---|---|---|
| Coexisting illness and risk factors. % |  |  |  |  |  |  |
| History of MI | 44.8 | 50.4 | 1.23 | 1 | 0.28 | n.s. |
| History of hypertension | 76.6 | 92.6 | 15.15 | 1 | 0.00 | ** |
| History of diabetes | 35.8 | 42.1 | 1.65 | 1 | 0.19 | n.s. |
| History of hypercholesterolemia | 68.6 | 74.4 | 1.54 | 1 | 0.22 | n.s. |
| History of renal failure | 17.5 | 18.5 | 0.058 | 1 | 0.81 | n.s. |
| History of previous PCI | 29.4 | 37.6 | 2.92 | 1 | 0.08 | + |
| Smoking % |  |  |  |  |  |  |
| No | 20.1 | 53.7 | 54.78 | 1 | 0.00 | ** |
| Previous | 59.6 | 34.7 | 23.92 | 1 | 0.00 | ** |
| Yes | 20.3 | 11.6 | 4.85 | 1 | 0.03 | * |

Note. n.s. non significant +p < 0.10 *p < 0.05 **p < 0.01

MI: Myocardial infarction

PCI: Percutaneous coronary intervention

**Intraoperative Data**

The rates of procedure priority and intraoperative complications as well as the average bypass time and time spent in the intensive care unit were similar in men and women. Overall, except for infections, intraoperative and postoperative complications appeared to be rare. More women than men experienced neurological complications, but rates of infarction, pneumothorax, infection and renal failure during this period of hospitalization were comparable to those of men (Table 10).

**Table 10. Gender Differences in Perioperative Characteristics: Significance of $\chi^2$-tests and t-tests**

|  | Men n= 458 | Women n= 121 | $\chi^2/t$ | df | p |  |
|---|---|---|---|---|---|---|
| **Procedure Priority %** |  |  |  |  |  |  |
| Elective | 26.4 | 26.4 | 0.00 | 1 | 0.99 | n.s. |
| Urgent | 24.0 | 24.8 | 0.03 | 1 | 0.86 | n.s. |
| Emergency / Salvage | 1.3 | 1.7 | 0.08 | 1 | 0.77 | n.s. |
| **Bypass Time (min.) M±SD** | 116.20 ± 58.74 | 110.43 ± 60.59 | 0.92 | 541 | 0.36 | n.s. |
| **Intensive Care Unit (days) M±SD** | 2.23 ± 3.47 | 2.78 ± 4.64 | -1.42 | 577 | 0.16 | n.s. |
| **Intraoperative Complications %** | 2.4 | 2.3 | 1.29 | 3 | 0.73 | n.s. |
| **Postoperative Complications %** |  |  |  |  |  |  |
| Infarction | 3.5 | 2.5 | 0.31 | 1 | 0.58 | n.s. |
| Pneumothrax | 4.1 | 4.1 | 0.00 | 1 | 0.99 | n.s. |
| Neurological complications | 1.7 | 5.0 | 4.19 | 1 | 0.04 | * |
| Infection | 28.6 | 28.1 | 1.09 | 6 | 0.98 | n.s. |
| Renal failure | 2.0 | 2.5 | 0.13 | 1 | 0.72 | n.s. |

Note. n.s. non significant *p < 0.05

**Completeness of Revascularization**

Table 11 shows the gender comparison of the distribution of diseased and grafted vessels. More men than women had triple-vessel disease, whereas more women had double-vessel disease. The rate of patients with left main stenosis did not differ significantly between men and women. With regard to the distribution of vessels grafted, the pattern seems similar to the pattern of diseased vessels with one exception: women were more than twice as likely as men to receive only one graft.

The question of whether women bear a greater risk of incomplete revascularization was addressed by calculating the ratio of diseased vessels to vessels grafted. The revascularization status was obtained by calculating the ratio of diseased vessels and vessels grafted. The fact that left main stem stenosis usually requires two bypasses was accounted for in this calculation. If the number of diseased vessels corresponded exactly to the number of vessels grafted, then the resulting coefficient should be less than or equal to 1. Otherwise, if the coefficient exceeded 1, this might point to incomplete revascularization. Table 11 shows that the coefficient was ≥ 1 in 14% of men and almost 25% of women. Thus, in accordance with the assumption, the rate of incomplete revascularization was higher in women than in men.

**Table 11. Number of Vessels Diseased, Vessels Grafted, Significance of $\chi^2$-tests**

|  | Men n= 458 | Women n= 121 | $\chi^2$ | df | p |  |
|---|---|---|---|---|---|---|
| 1-vessel disease % | 6.3 | 9.1 | 1.13 | 1 | 0.29 | n.s. |
| 2-vessel disease % | 12.2 | 25.6 | 13.45 | 1 | 0.001 | ** |
| 3-vessel disease % | 68.8 | 51.2 | 12.96 | 1 | 0.001 | ** |
| Left main (coronary artery) stenosis % | 12.2 | 14.0 | 0.29 | 1 | 0.59 | n.s. |
| Grafts % |  |  |  |  |  |  |
| 1 | 8.1 | 16.5 | 7.70 | 1 | 0.01 | ** |
| 2 | 17.5 | 29.8 | 9.02 | 1 | 0.01 | ** |
| ≥3 | 72.9 | 50.4 | 22.38 | 1 | 0.001 | ** |
| Revascularization (%) |  |  |  |  |  |  |
| ≥1= Incomplete | 14.2 | 24.8 | 7.84 | 1 | 0.005 | ** |

Note. n.s. non significant **p < 0.01

## Risk Scores

As part of the present study, a multitude of risk factors has been assessed. In order to reduce the total number of variables, two risk scores, the EuroSCORE (Nashef et al., 1999) and the Framingham Score (Wilson et al., 1998), have been calculated. Both risk scores include special weightings for age. Age is, on the one hand, a clinical risk factor and on the other hand a sociodemographic factor, which is associated with a multitude of psychological variables. Therefore, both risk scores were first calculated including age. In a second calculation, age was excluded.

## The EuroSCORE

The EuroSCORE includes some patient-related factors, some factors derived from the preoperative status, and factors depending on the timing and nature of the operation. Detailed representations of weights and analyses of gender differences in the respective risk factors are shown in Table 12.

**Table 12. EuroSCORE Risk Factors by Gender: Significance of $\chi^2$-tests and t-tests**

| Risk factors | Score | Men n= 458 | Women n= 121 | $\chi^2/t$ | df | p | |
|---|---|---|---|---|---|---|---|
| **Age groups (%)** | | | | | | | |
| 1. <61 | (0) | 24.7 | 14.0 | 6.20 | 1 | 0.013 | ** |
| 2. 61-65 | (1) | 25.8 | 12.4 | 9.67 | 1 | 0.002 | *** |
| 3. 66-70 | (2) | 24.5 | 17.4 | 2.73 | 1 | 0.099 | + |
| 4. 71-75 | (3) | 12.9 | 24.8 | 10.44 | 1 | 0.001 | *** |
| 5. 76-80 | (4) | 8.7 | 20.7 | 13.66 | 1 | 0.000 | *** |
| 6. 81-85 | (5) | 3.5 | 7.4 | 3.61 | 1 | 0.06 | + |
| 7.>86 | (6) | 0 | 3.3 | 15.25 | 1 | 0.000 | *** |
| Female sex | (2) | | | | | | |
| Extracardiac arteriopathy (%) | (2) | 24.5 | 28.1 | 0.67 | 1 | 0.41 | n.s. |
| Renal failure (creatinine>200μmol/L) | (2) | 1.3 | 5.8 | 8.73 | 1 | 0.003 | ** |
| Operative incidence (redo) (%) | (3) | 6.6 | 6.6 | 0.00 | 1 | 0.98 | n.s. |
| Active endocarditis (%) | (3) | 0.0 | 0.0 | --- | --- | --- | n.s. |
| Critical preoperative state (%) | (3) | 0.0 | 0.8 | 3.79 | 1 | 0.05 | * |
| Unstable angina (NYHA= 4) (%) | (2) | 0.2 | 2.5 | 7.13 | 1 | 0.008 | ** |
| EF[a] <30% (%) | (3) | 7 | 6.6 | 0.02 | 1 | 0.885 | n.s. |
| EF 30-50% (%) | (1) | 32.8 | 31.4 | 0.08 | 1 | 0.779 | n.s. |
| EF>50% (%) | (0) | 60.3 | 62.0 | 0.12 | 1 | 0.73 | n.s. |
| Pulmonary hypertension (%) | (2) | 1.3 | 1.7 | 0.08 | 1 | 0.774 | n.s. |
| Operative status: emergency (%) | (2) | 1.7 | 1.7 | 0.01 | 1 | 0.944 | n.s. |
| Other than isolated CABG (%) | (2) | 0.2 | 0.0 | 0.27 | 1 | 0.607 | n.s. |
| Surgery on thoracic aorta (%) | (3) | 0.0 | 0.0 | --- | --- | --- | n.s. |
| Postoperative infarction (%) | (4) | 3.5 | 2.5 | 0.31 | 1 | 0.578 | n.s. |

Notes. n.s. non significant +p < 0.10 *p < 0.05 **p < 0.01 ***p < 0.001

[a] Ejection Fraction

Men and women differed on several dimensions of the EuroSCORE. Women were older than men; they were significantly more likely to experience unstable angina pectoris, renal failure (creatinine > 200μmol/L) and a critical preoperative state (Table 12). In order to avoid a bias in gender comparison, the risk weight for female gender was excluded from the calculation. However, even after the elimination of female sex, women had higher scores on the EuroSCORE ($M_{men}$ = 3.12 ± 2.2; $M_{women}$ = 4.24 ± 2.5; t (577) = -4.84, p < 0.001). Three risk categories indicate the severity of risk. A greater proportion of women than men fell into the high-risk category, and, correspondingly, more men than women fell into the lowest risk category (Table 13). When age was eliminated from the analyses, the gender difference in the sumscore was no longer significant ($M_{men}$ = 1.46 ± 1.63; $M_{women}$ = 1.63 ± 1.86; t (577) = -0.98, n.s.). Thus, age is an important factor for the comparison of men and women.

**Table 13. EuroSCORE[a] Means and Risk Categories: Significance of $\chi^2$-tests**

|  | Men<br>n= 458 | Women<br>n= 121 | $\chi^2$ | df | p |  |
|---|---|---|---|---|---|---|
| Risk Categories (%) |  |  |  |  |  |  |
| Low risk (0-2) | 42.4 | 22.3 | 16.29 | 1 | 0.001 | *** |
| Medium risk (3-5) | 42.8 | 52.1 | 3.33 | 1 | 0.07 | + |
| High risk (≥6) | 14.8 | 25.6 | 7.836 | 1 | 0.005 | ** |

Notes. +p < 0.10 **p < 0.01 ***p < 0.001

(a) female gender excluded from the EuroSCORE

**The Framingham Score**

While the EuroSCORE is confined to baseline health characteristics and perioperative complications, the Framingham Score has its main focus on common risk factors such as age, cholesterol, blood pressure, cigarette smoking and diabetes mellitus (Table 14). Apart from age, more women than men had high cholesterol levels and hypertension, whereas men were more often smokers. Overall, women scored higher on the Framingham Score than men ($M_{men}$ = 8.5 ± 2.86; $M_{women}$ = 10.61 ± 3.44; t (577) = -6.91, p < 0.001). Age was excluded from the Framingham Score for the same reasons as those described above for the EuroSCORE. When age was excluded from the calculation of the Framingham Score, the gender difference in the mean score diminished and no longer reached significance ($M_{men}$ = 3.04 ± 2.53; $M_{women}$ = 2.87 ± 3.15; t (577) = .64, n.s.).

**Table 14. Framingham Score Risk factors by Gender: Significance of $\chi^2$-tests**

| Risk factors | Score Men | Score Women | Men n= 458 | Women n= 121 | $\chi^2$ | df | p | |
|---|---|---|---|---|---|---|---|---|
| Age groups (%) | | | | | | | | |
| 1. <39 | 0 | -4 | 0.4 | 0.0 | 0.53[a] | 1 | 1.00 | n.s. |
| 2. 40-44 | 1 | 0 | 1.7 | 0.8 | 0.53[a] | 1 | 0.47 | n.s. |
| 3. 45-49 | 2 | 3 | 1.7 | 0.8 | 0.53[a] | 1 | 0.69 | n.s. |
| 4. 50-54 | 3 | 6 | 7.6 | 3.3 | 2.87 | 1 | 0.10 | + |
| 5. 55-59 | 4 | 7 | 10.9 | 8.3 | 0.73 | 1 | 0.39 | n.s. |
| 6. 60-64 | 5 | 8 | 21.0 | 10.7 | 6.54 | 1 | 0.01 | * |
| 7. 65-69 | 6 | 8 | 26.6 | 18.2 | 3.66 | 1 | 0.06 | + |
| 8. >70 | 7 | 8 | 29.9 | 57.9 | 32.53 | 1 | 0.000 | *** |
| Cholesterol (%) | | | | | | | | |
| <160 | -3 | -3 | 23.6 | 14.9 | 4.26 | 1 | 0.04 | * |
| 160-199 | 0 | 0 | 33.4 | 43.0 | 3.83 | 1 | 0.05 | * |
| 200-239 | 1 | 1 | 29.7 | 30.6 | 0.04 | 1 | 0.85 | n.s. |
| 240-279 | 2 | 2 | 10.7 | 8.3 | 0.62 | 1 | 0.43 | n.s. |
| >280 | 3 | 3 | 2.6 | 3.3 | 0.18 | 1 | 0.68 | n.s. |
| Hypertension (%) | | | | | | | | |
| <120 | 0 | -3 | 32.8 | 28.1 | 0.96 | 1 | 0.33 | n.s. |
| 120-129 | 0 | 0 | 19.7 | 14.9 | 1.44 | 1 | 0.23 | n.s. |
| 130-139 | 1 | 0 | 25.8 | 14.9 | 6.31 | 1 | 0.012 | * |
| 140-159 | 2 | 2 | 23.8 | 32.2 | 3.58 | 1 | 0.06 | + |
| >160 | 3 | 3 | 4.4 | 9.9 | 5.65 | 1 | 0.017 | * |
| Smoker (%) | 2 | 2 | 79.9 | 46.3 | 54.78 | 1 | 0.00 | ** |
| Diabetes (%) | 2 | 4 | 35.8 | 42.1 | 1.65 | 1 | 0.19 | n.s. |

Notes. n.s. non significant +p < 0.10 *p < 0.05 **p < 0.01 ***p < 0.001

(a) exact test according to Fisher with at least one cell displaying a frequency of < 5

## Psychosocial Factors

It was hypothesized that women were more anxious and depressive before surgery. In accordance with this hypothesis, the t-test for independent samples revealed marked gender differences in depression and anxiety (Table 15). Women were more anxious and displayed higher levels of depression before surgery. Anxiety and depression were strongly related in both men and in women ($r_{men} = 0.60$, p < 0.001; $r_{women} = 0.72$, p < 0.001). However, the correlation between anxiety and depression was stronger in women: the correlation coefficients of men and women differed significantly in their absolute size (p < 0.05).

**Table 15. Gender Differences in Depression and Anxiety: Significance of t-tests for Unpaired Samples**

|  | Men= 458 | | Women= 121 | | | | |
|---|---|---|---|---|---|---|---|
|  | M | SD | M | SD | t | df | p |
| Anxiety | 5.63 | 3.79 | 7.02 | 3.91 | -3.47 | 574 | 0.001 |
| Depression[a] | 5.97 | 4.52 | 8.17 | 5.36 | -4.58 | 576 | 0.001 |
| Social support[a] | 21.41 | 4.16 | 20.65 | 4.53 | 1.65[b] | 175.59 | 0.10 |

Note.

(a) The test of significance was performed on square root transformed data – nonetheless, to facilitate the interpretation, the table displays the untransformed data

(b) Equal variances not assumed ($p < 0.05$)

HADS Hospital Anxiety and Depression Scale: Range 0-21; PHQ Patient Health Questionnaire: Range 0-27; Social Support: Range 0-25. Higher values indicate higher anxiety, higher depression and more social support.

Women were older than men, had a lower education level and were more likely to live alone. Preoperatively women had higher levels of depression and anxiety. They had more often a history of hypertension and a history of previous PCI, whereas men were more likely to be smokers. After surgery, women more often experienced neurological complications than men. Men more often had triple-vessel disease, but also received more grafts than women. However, the rate of incomplete revascularization was higher in women. Established risk scores reflected the risk profiles of men and women, with age being the dominant risk factor for women.

### 4.1.2 Predicting Mortality

An analysis of mortality using the $\chi^2$-test yielded a marked gender difference in mortality, with 15 of 121 female patients (12.4%) dying within 1 year after surgery compared to 24 of 458 male patients (5.2%) ($\chi^2 = 7.80$, $p < .01$). Thus, women were more than twice as likely to die during the first year after CABG as men (RR = 2.26). This result is consistent with the assumption that gender is a predictor for mortality after bypass surgery. Do sociodemographic and psychosocial variables – in addition to clinical parameters – make significant contributions to the explanation of the gender difference in mortality? The following sections deal with this question, which alludes to one of the central topics of the present study.

### Single Relationships between Risk Factors and Mortality

In order to examine the interplay of different risk factors and to extract the most meaningful ones, the first step of analysis included an examination of single correlations of risk factors with mortality. Table 16 shows φ-coefficients for categorical data and Pearson's r-coefficient for continuous data.

**Table 16. Associations between Risk factors and Mortality: Significance of φ [d] and Pearson's Correlations**

| | Entire sample N= 579 | | Men n= 458 | | Women n= 121 | |
|---|---|---|---|---|---|---|
| | φ[d] / r | p | φ[d] / r | p | φ[d] / r | p |
| Female gender | 0.12 | ** | | | | |
| Age | 0.12 | ** | 0.11 | * | 0.08 | n.s. |
| Education level[f] | 0.13 | ** | 0.05 | n.s. | 0.19 | * |
| Partner status | 0.02 | n.s. | -0.06 | n.s. | -0.05 | n.s. |
| Social support | 0.08 | + | 0.08 | +[a] | 0.11 | n.s. |
| Anxiety | 0.06 | 0.12 | 0.01 | n.s. | 0.14 | n.s. |
| Depression | 0.11 | ** | 0.08 | n.s. | 0.15 | + |
| Congestive heart failure | 0.15 | *** | 0.11 | * | 0.22 | * |
| LVEF | -0.17 | ** | -0.09[e] | * | -0.43 | ** |
| Prior infarction | 0.10 | * | 0.12 | ** | 0.02 | n.s. |
| Hypertension | 0.01 | n.s. | 0.04[e] | n.s. | -0.18 | n.s. |
| Diabetes | 0.08 | + | 0.03 | n.s. | 0.19 | * |
| Hyperlipidemia | -0.09 | * | -0.01[e] | n.s. | -0.35 | **[a] |
| Renal dysfunction | 0.04 | n.s. | -0.01 | n.s.[a] | 0.08 | n.s.[a] |
| Smoking | -0.02 | n.s. | 0.07 | n.s.[a] | -0.10 | n.s. |
| BMI>30 | -0.03 | n.s. | 0.01 | n.s. | -0.11 | n.s.[a] |
| Framingham Score[b] | 0.02 | n.s. | 0.03 | n.s. | 0.02 | n.s. |
| Operative status: Emergency | 0.09 | + | 0.06 | n.s. | 0.15 | n.s.[a] |
| Post Op Factors | | | | | | |
| Infarction | 0.22 | *** | 0.22 | **[a] | 0.26 | +[a] |
| Pneumothorax | 0.05 | n.s. | 0.09 | +[a] | -0.08 | n.s.[a] |
| Cerebrovascular event | 0.05 | n.s. | 0.04 | n.s.[a] | 0.03 | n.s.[a] |
| Kidney failure | 0.15 | ** | 0.11 | +[a] | 0.26 | *[a] |
| Complications | 0.22 | ** | 0.23 | ** | 0.21 | +[a] |
| Incomplete revascularization | 0.07 | + | -0.01[e] | n.s. | 0.19 | * |
| EuroSCORE[c] | 0.32 | *** | 0.24[e] | *** | 0.44 | *** |

Notes. n.s. non significant $+p < 0.10$ $*p < 0.05$ $**p < 0.01$ $***p < 0.001$

(a) Fisher's exact test with at least one cell below 5

(b) Framingham Score: age excluded

(c) EuroSCORE: age excluded

(d) The phi coefficient (φ) is a measure of the degree of association between two binary variables and similar to the correlation coefficient in its interpretation

(e) Gender difference in size of correlation coefficients (significance of either Fisher's Z-transformation or Breslow-Day-test). All correlations in this table are tested for gender differences. Grey marked cells indicate significant differences (for descriptive purposes without alpha-error adjustment).

(f) no vocational training

The φ-coefficient is a measure of the degree of association between two binary variables and is similar to the r-coefficient in its interpretation. Therefore, both coefficients are summarized in one table. Not only gender, but also age, education level, depression, congestive heart failure, LVEF, prior infarction, diabetes, hyperlipidemia, postoperative infarction and postoperative complications reached significance in the entire sample. Not all predictors reached significance in men *and* women. Whereas prior infarction and age were significantly related to mortality in the male sample, the same was true for diabetes, incomplete revascularization, depression and a low education level only in the female sample.

One assumption was that risk factors might differ in the strength of influence on mortality between men and women. For example, if the correlation between age and mortality is r = 0.11 in men and r = 0.08 in women, it is of interest to know whether the difference between these two correlation coefficients is significant. Using the Fisher r-to-z transformation, the significance of differences between two correlation coefficients was tested for continuous data. The outcome of this test depends not only on the size of the total difference between the two coefficients, but also on the size of the samples and on the size of the coefficients themselves. In general, due to the fact that the reliability of the correlation coefficient increases with its absolute value, relatively small differences between *large* correlation coefficients can be significant, whereas the same difference between *small* correlations may not reach significance. The Breslow-Day test was applied for categorical data. In accordance with the initial assumption, men and women differed on some risk factors, the differences being more marked in women than in men. This was true for LVEF, hypertension, hyperlipidemia, incomplete revascularization and the EuroSCORE (respective cells marked grey).

### *Interactions Between Gender and Risk Factors*

In the previous section, it has been shown that risk factors contribute differently to mortality in men and women. Because this could point to moderator effects, further analyses with interaction terms were conducted. A moderator is a variable that affects the correlation between two other variables (Figure 3). For example, hyperlipidemia was significantly correlated with mortality in women, but not in men. In this case, gender might moderate the effect of hyperlipidemia on mortality.

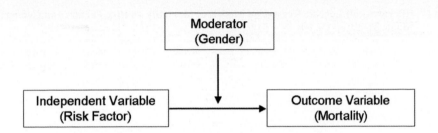

*Figure 3. Moderator Model According to Baron and Kenny (1986)*

To test the significance of gender as a moderator, the following planned multiple regression models, including single interaction terms, were tested:

*Mortality = gender + risk factor + gender * risk factor.*

Included were the following risk factors: diabetes, hyperlipidemia, smoking, hypertension, LVEF, EuroSCORE, low education level and partner status. None of the interaction models reached significance at the $p < 0.05$ level.

**Multiple Correlations with Mortality**

Does gender remain an independent risk factor for mortality after adjustment for psychosocial and somatic risk factors? To answer this question, all risk factors for mortality, which reached significance in either men *or* women at a level of $p < 0.05$ (see Table 16, previous chapter) were selected a priori: this was true, apart from gender, also for age, education, depression, LVEF, prior infarction, congestive heart failure, incomplete revascularization, and diabetes. The EuroSCORE, which proved to be highly significant for both genders, includes all postoperative complications that are listed in Table 16. Because each complication appeared to be rare (see Table 10), the EuroSCORE as an established sumscore was used instead.

The main effect of gender on mortality was highly significant (OR = 2.56; 95%CI = 1.30-5.05; $p < 0.01$). Using SPSS REGRESSION, single mediator models were calculated with the a priori selected variables entering in the first step, whereas gender was included in the second step (Table 17). The last column in Table 17 shows how the influence of gender on mortality diminishes after adjustment for the respective single risk factors.

**Table 17. (Hierarchical) Logistic Regression Models of Mortality on Risk Factors and Gender: Single Mediator Models (N = 579)**

| Variable | Model 1 OR(CI) | Model 2 OR(CI) | Model 3 OR(CI) | Model 4 OR(CI) | Model 5 OR(CI) | Model 6 OR(CI) | Model 7 OR(CI) | Model 8 OR(CI) | Model 9 OR(CI) |
|---|---|---|---|---|---|---|---|---|---|
| Age | 1.06(1.02-1.10)** | | | | | | | | |
| Education level (1) No voc.training | | 3.67(1.17-11.5)** | | | | | | | |
| (2) Apprenticeship | | 1.58(0.63-3.95) n.s. | | | | | | | |
| Depression[a] | | | 1.54(1.09-2.16)** | | | | | | |
| Heart Failure | | | | 3.11(1.61-6.01)*** | | | | | |
| LVEF | | | | | 0.95(0.93-0.98)*** | | | | |
| Diabetes | | | | | | 1.86(0.97-3.58)+ | | | |
| Prior infarction | | | | | | | 2.22(1.13-4.36)* | | |
| Revascularization | | | | | | | | 0.50(0.24-1.05)+ | |
| EuroSCORE[b] | | | | | | | | | 1.70(1.43-2.01)*** |
| Gender [c] (second step) | 2.01 (0.98-0.09)+ | 2.00 (0.94-0.10)+ | 2.3(1.14-4.65)* | 2.36(1.19-4.72)** | 2.4(1.18-4.89)** | 2.48(1.25-4.90)** | 2.48(1.25-4.91)** | 2.4(1.21-4.77)** | 2.42(1.17-5.03)** |

Notes. +p < 0.10 *p < 0.05 **p < 0.01 ***p < 0.001

(a) square root transformation

(b) EuroSCORE: age excluded

(c) OR of gender after adjustment for the respective risk factor

A model predictive of mortality was built to examine the mutual interplay of all risk factors and their influence on 1-year mortality. Using SPSS REGRESSION, multiple logistic regression analyses were performed on mortality. The process started by forcing in gender, age, education, depression, heart failure, LVEF, prior infarction, diabetes, incomplete revascularization and the modified EuroSCORE. Backward stepwise selection was employed to build a final model (Table 18). Thereby the least significant variables were dropped, as long as they were not significant at the chosen level (i.e. p > 0.10). This process was continued by successively refitting reduced models and applying the same rule until all remaining variables were statistically significant. Table 18 shows the results of these analyses. Gender as a predictor was no longer significant in the final model after adjustment for all risk factors. Education, prior infarction, diabetes and heart failure were eliminated from the final model.

**Table 18. Final Model: Predicting Mortality in the Entire Sample: Results of Logistic Regression Analysis (Backward Elimination)**

|  | Final Model N= 579 | | |
| --- | --- | --- | --- |
|  | OR | CI (95%) | p |
| Age | 1.05 | 1.01-1.10 | * |
| Depression[a] | 1.50 | 1.03-2.19 | * |
| EuroSCORE[b] | 1.71 | 1.43-2.04 | *** |

Notes. +p < 0.05 *p < 0.05 **p < 0.01 ***p < 0.001

(a) square root transformation

(b) age excluded

However, it is noteworthy that it was not one single risk factor that could fully explain the association between gender and mortality but rather a combination of the nine variables apart from gender. In order to support this conclusion, the residual score, which is the difference between the observed value and the value predicted by the model, was calculated post hoc. If the proposed model could explain the gender difference in mortality in this sample, the association between the residual score and gender would not be significant. Indeed, the correlation between the residual score and gender was negligible (r = 0.04, n.s.).

One empirical prediction of this study was that the relationship between gender and mortality is mediated by psychosocial and clinical risk factors. As described above (section 4.1.1), women indeed had a lower educational status and a less favourable risk profile. According to Baron and Kenny (1986), four requirements must be fulfilled in order to statistically support the assumption of mediation: (1) the association between the independent variable (gender) and the mediators (risk factors) must be significant; (2) there must be a significant association between the independent variable (gender) and the dependent variable (mortality); (3) when the dependent variable (mortality) is regressed on both the independent variable (gender) and the mediators (risk factors), there must be a significant effect of the mediator on the dependent variable (mortality); (4) if all three conditions described above were true, then the effect of gender on mortality would be expected to be reduced in the third compared to the second condition (see Figure 4).

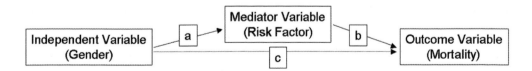

*Figure 4. The Mediator Model, Modified after Baron and Kenny (1986)*

As shown in the previous sections, the first of Baron and Kenny's requirements (path a in Figure 4) is fulfilled: there is a significant association between gender and the risk factors included in the regression analysis (age, education, depression, EuroSCORE). The second requirement (path c) is also fulfilled: the association between gender and mortality is highly significant. The third requirement was tested within the regression analysis (Table 18). After adjustment for all risk factors, the association between gender and mortality diminished (fourth requirement). Single analyses including sex and the respective risk factor revealed that the association diminished, but remained significant if depression, EuroSCORE, prior infarction, diabetes, revascularization, LVEF or heart failure were controlled for, but became non-significant once age or education was included.

Not only gender but also age, education, depression, heart failure, LVEF, diabetes, prior infarction, incomplete revascularization and the modified EuroSCORE were related to mortality in the entire sample. After adjustment for all risk factors, gender was no longer an independent predictor for mortality. The EuroSCORE, depression and age were the dominant predictors for mortality in the entire sample, whereas education and age were the main mediators for the relationship between gender and mortality. Overall, there is sufficient statistical support for the mediation hypotheses that the relationship between gender and mortality is mediated by sociodemographic, psychosocial and clinical risk factors. With respect to the moderator hypotheses, none of the interaction terms reached significance. However, there was a trend for risk factors being more strongly related to mortality in women than in men.

### 4.1.3 Predicting Physical Functioning

Physical functioning reflects the subjective health status of patients. In both men and women, physical functioning differed markedly from that of the German norm aged 60-70 years (*SF-36 health survey manual,* Bullinger and Kirchberger, 1998). On a scale that ranged from 0 to 100, CABG patients displayed scores that fell on average 22 points below the scores of the norm sample (Figure 5). Notably, in the younger age group the difference between female CABG patients and women of the norm population was large (28.5 points). The gender difference in the population of CABG patients was highly significant, with women displaying lower values than men ($M_{men} = 54.16 \pm 26.40$; $M_{women} = 40.83 \pm 25.61$; t (577) = 4.97, p < 0.001).

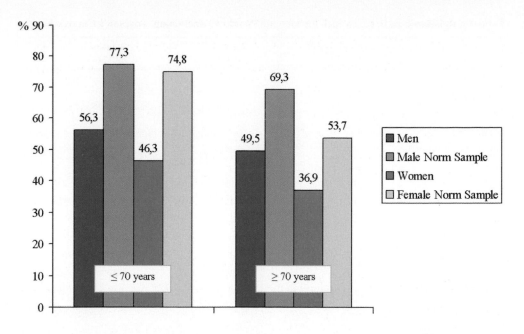

*Figure 5. Physical Functioning: Comparison with the German Norm Sample by Gender and Age*

Following the procedure described in section 4.1.2, a final model was constructed to identify the most meaningful predictors for physical functioning. First, physical functioning was correlated with the same predictors as mortality. Second, possible interactions were analyzed and, if significantly correlated with physical functioning at a $p < 0.05$ level, included in the regression equation. Since in this context preoperative physical functioning was the outcome parameter, only preoperative predictors were included in the analyses. Consequently, postoperative parameters (e.g. postoperative infarction or active endocarditis) were also excluded from the EuroSCORE.

**Single Relationships Between Risk Factors and Physical Functioning**

A variety of risk factors significantly correlated with physical functioning (Table 19). This was true, apart from gender, for age, education, partner status, social support, anxiety, depression, congestive heart failure, renal failure, BMI, LVEF and the modified EuroSCORE. To test whether gender differences in correlation coefficients differed, all possible pairs of coefficients were tested. None of the differences between two correlation coefficients, $r_{men}$ and $r_{women}$ reached significance. In other words, the correlations between physical functioning and risk factors in men did not differ from the correlations between physical functioning and risk factors in women.

**Table 19. Relationships Between Risk Factors and Physical Functioning: Pearson's Correlations**

| | Entire sample N= 579 | | Men n= 458 | | Women n= 121 | |
|---|---|---|---|---|---|---|
| Risk Factors | r | p | r | p | r | p |
| Female Gender | 0.20 | *** | | | | |
| Age | -0.17 | *** | -0.11 | * | -0.20 | * |
| Education level | 0.23 | *** | 0.20 | *** | 0.16 | + |
| Partner Status (with partner) | -0.18 | *** | -0.08 | n.s. | -0.19 | * |
| Social support | 0.13 | ** | 0.15 | *** | 0.01 | n.s. |
| Anxiety | -0.20 | *** | -0.19 | *** | -0.14 | n.s. |
| Depression[(c)] | -0.42 | *** | -0.42 | *** | -0.31 | *** |
| Congestive Heart failure | -0.24 | *** | -0.21 | *** | -0.32 | *** |
| LVEF | 0.18 | *** | 0.15 | *** | 0.27 | *** |
| Prior infarction | -0.07 | n.s. | -0.07 | n.s. | -0.05 | n.s. |
| Hypertension | -0.05 | n.s. | -0.02 | n.s. | 0.00 | n.s. |
| Diabetes | -0.02 | n.s. | 0.00 | n.s. | -0.06 | n.s. |
| Hyperlipidemia | -0.07 | n.s. | 0.11 | * | -0.03 | n.s. |
| Renal dysfunction | -0.17 | ** | -0.18 | ** | -0.14 | n.s. |
| Smoking | -0.01 | n.s. | -0.11 | ** | 0.01 | n.s. |
| BMI | -0.12 | ** | -0.15 | *** | -0.11 | n.s. |
| Framingham SCORE[(a)] | -0.06 | n.s. | -0.05 | n.s. | -0.11 | n.s. |
| Operative status (emergent) | -0.04 | n.s. | -0.03 | n.s. | -0.09 | n.s. |
| EuroSCORE [(a) (b)] | -0.26 | *** | -0.23 | *** | -0.14 | n.s. |

Notes. $+p < 0.05$ $*p < 0.05$ $**p < 0.01$ $***p < 0.001$

(a) Age excluded

(b) Postoperative parameters excluded

(c) square root transformed variable

### Interactions Between Gender and Risk Factors

Next, interactions between gender and risk factors were tested. Using SPSS REGRESSION, multiple regression analyses were conducted to test the following model (see section 4.1.2 for a more detailed description of the moderator model):

*Physical functioning = Gender + Risk factor + Gender * Risk factor.*

With regard to physical functioning, none of the interaction terms reached significance, indicating that risk factors are not differently associated with physical functioning in men and women. In other words, gender does not moderate the relationship between risk factors and physical functioning in this analysis.

## Multiple Correlations with Physical Functioning

In the two previous sections, simple associations between risk factors and physical functioning as well as the respective interactions have been tested. All risk factors, which were significant in either men or women at the $p < 0.05$ level were selected for inclusion in the regression model. Thus, gender, age, education, partner status, social support, anxiety, depression, congestive heart failure, renal failure, BMI, LVEF, and the EuroSCORE were included. Because none of the interaction terms reached significance, more parsimonious models without interactions were run.

**Table 20. Predicting Physical functioning[a] in the Entire Sample: Results of Linear Multiple Regression Analysis (Backward Elimination) (N = 579)**

|  | SE | β | p |
|---|---|---|---|
| Gender | 2.65 | -0.07 | + |
| Age | 0.12 | -0.18 | *** |
| Education | 1.84 | 0.10 | * |
| BMI | 0.25 | -0.13 | *** |
| Depression [b] | 1.07 | -0.36 | *** |
| Renal failure | 2.69 | -0.08 | * |
| Heart failure | 2.20 | -0.16 | *** |

Notes. $+p < 0.05$ $*p < 0.05$ $**p < 0.01$ $***p < 0.001$

(a) Higher values display better Physical Functioning (range: 0-100)

(b) Square root transformed variable

Using SPSS LINEAR REGRESSION with backward elimination, a model with the most meaningful predictors was constructed. Seven risk factors remained in the final model (see Table 20): gender, age, education, BMI, depression, heart failure and renal failure. However, the significance of gender was only marginal ($p < 0.10$) after adjustment for other risk factors. The strongest predictor in this analysis was depression ($\beta = -0.36$). Overall, there is statistical support for the hypothesis that the relationship of gender and physical functioning is partially mediated by risk factors. However, post hoc analyses with single regression analyses (including gender and the respective risk factor) revealed that none of the risk factors alone mediated the relationship between gender and physical functioning. In other words, if the respective risk factor was entered into the analysis, gender still remained significant. In accordance to the procedure of the gender/mortality analysis, the residual score of all risk factors, which had been included in the regression analysis was calculated and were subsequently correlated with gender. The resulting coefficient was $r = 0.07$, $p = 0.13$ indicating that all risk factors together explained most of the variance of the gender / physical functioning relationship.

A multitude of risk factors were associated with physical functioning. After adjusting for all risk factors, the predictive power of gender diminished and was then only marginally significant. Age, low education level, BMI, depression, renal failure and heart failure turned out to be the dominant risk factors for physical functioning. Neither the Framingham Score nor the EuroSCORE remained in the final model.

*Comparing the Two Outcome Parameters*

The relationship between physical functioning before surgery and 1-year-mortality was weak in the entire sample ($r = -0.10$, n.s.). In men, the correlation between physical functioning and mortality did not reach significance ($r_{men} = -0.05$, n.s.), whereas in women the association was significant ($r_{women} = -0.18$, $p < 0.05$). In contrast to the regression on mortality (section 4.1.2), education remained a significant predictor for physical functioning after adjustment for other risk factors. The BMI, which, in contrast to physical functioning, was not significantly associated with mortality and thus not included in the respective regression analysis, proved to be a significant predictor for physical functioning in the final model. With respect to mortality, the EuroSCORE proved to be the strongest predictor. For physical functioning, the dominant predictor was depression. Gender as a predictor for physical functioning remained in the final model, but with only marginal significance at the $p < 0.10$ level.

After surgery, the relative risk of 1-year mortality among women exceeded the mortality rate of men more than twofold. Age, depression and the risk factors summarized in the EuroSCORE were the major predictors for mortality in the entire sample. Women displayed a markedly lower physical functioning than men shortly before CABG surgery. Age, depression, education, BMI, renal failure and heart failure were the dominant predictors for physical functioning. Gender no longer remained an independent risk factor for either physical functioning or mortality after adjustment for psychosocial and clinical risk factors.

## 4.2 Predictors of Well-Being Based on Longitudinal Data

*Do clinical parameters and stress due to domestic tasks affect depression and physical functioning after surgery differently in men and women? How is depression related to physical functioning in the long term?* In this part of the results, analyses of the continuer sample over the three measurement points are presented, focussing on subjective parameters such as depression and stress due to housework after the operation. The measurement points of the longitudinal study are referred to as "T1" (1-2 days prior to surgery), "T2" (2 months after surgery) and "T3" (1 year after surgery).

As demonstrated in section 3.4.2, the full sample at T1 differed from the longitudinal sample with respect to some psychosocial and clinical variables. The drop-out and its consequences for the most important variables have been the focus of interest in the methods chapter. Socidemographic and clinical data have been investigated in detail in section 4.1.1. In the following section only those variables that are essential for the analysis of the longitudinal data are described again.

## 4.2.1 Description of Predictors

This section deals with a gender comparison of the psychosocial and clinical profiles using simple t-tests for continuous and $\chi^2$-tests for categorical data.

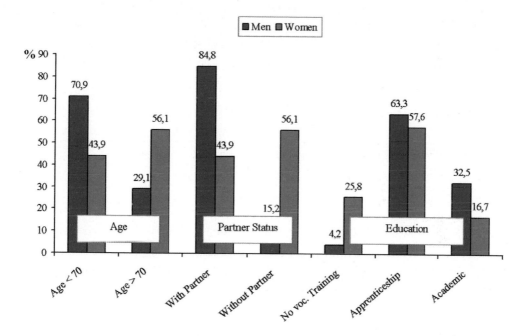

*Figure 6. Sociodemographic Characteristics by Gender: The Continuer Sample*

**Demographic and Social Factors**

The structure of the socio-economic data is described schematically in Figure 6. Women in the longitudinal sample were, on average, 3.4 years older than men ($M_{men} = 65.62 \pm 7.86$; $M_{women} = 69,06 \pm 9.49$; t (353) = -3.08, p < 0.05). In addition, 56% percent of women were over 70 years old compared to 29% of men ($\chi^2$ = 17.43; p < 0.001). Women were more likely to live alone or to be widowed ($\chi^2$ = 50.88; p < 0.001) and had a lower level of education ($\chi^2$ = 35.56; p < 0.001).

## Postoperative Depression and Anxiety

In this section, the course of depression and anxiety over the three measurement points is described. On a four-point scale, patients were asked to rate their symptoms of anxiety and depression. At all time points, women displayed higher anxiety scores than men. Means and standard deviations for the study variables are presented in Table 21.

**Table 21. Means and Standard Deviations of Physical Functioning by Gender**

|  | Men n= 289 | | Women n= 66 | |
|---|---|---|---|---|
|  | M | SD | M | SD |
| Depression T1 | 5.34 | 3.65 | 6.44 | 3.77 |
| Anxiety T1 | 4.97 | 3.58 | 6.44 | 3.75 |
| Social Support T1 | 21.16 | 4.09 | 21.03 | 4.18 |
| Depression T2 | 3.86 | 3.66 | 5.18 | 4.04 |
| Anxiety T2 | 4.67 | 3.98 | 6.03 | 4.39 |
| Social Support T2 | 22.15 | 4.05 | 20.91 | 4.56 |
| Depression T3 | 4.17 | 3.80 | 5.06 | 4.22 |
| Anxiety T3 | 4.42 | 4.02 | 5.33 | 4.42 |
| Social Support T3 | 21.87 | 4.23 | 20.68 | 5.03 |

Notes. Depression: Range from 0 to 27

Anxiety: Range from 0 to 21

Social support: Range from 5 to 25

Using SPSS GLM REPEATED MEASURES, a 2 (gender) by 3 (measurement points) repeated measures analysis of variance (ANOVAs) was conducted on all three variables.

The PHQ scores for depression were moderately skewed to the left with slight deviations from normality. Therefore all analyses requiring normal distributions were conducted both without and with square root transformations of PHQ scores at T1, T2 and T3, respectively. Given that the results did not vary substantially with regard to tests of significance, only results from transformed data are reported. Figure 7 shows the development of depression over time separated by gender. The analysis revealed a significant main effect for time ($F(2,349) = 4,341, p < 01$: $Eta^2 = 0.02$) and for the between-subjects factor gender ($F(1,349) = 4,699, p < 0.05$: $Eta^2 = 0.01$). With respect to anxiety, the analysis yielded a significant main effect for time ($F(2,602) = 22,16, p < 0.01$: $Eta^2 = 0.06$) and a significant main effect for gender (men versus women: $F(1,351) = 6,61, p < 0.01$: $Eta^2 = 0.02$). Concerning social support, the main effect for time was not significant. Post-hoc Bonferroni adjusted analyses revealed that men received more support than women two months after surgery ($t(1,349) = 2.11$, $p < 0.05$). Neither in anxiety and depression nor social support did the interaction terms reach significance. This means that though men and women differed in their baseline levels on these three variables, the improvement over time was similar in both genders.

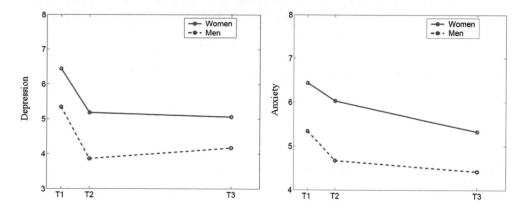

*Figure 7. Mean Level Changes in Depression and Anxiety by Gender*

Note (Depression): Higher values indicate higher depression (Range 0 - 27)

Note (Anxiety): Higher values indicate higher anxiety (Range 0 – 21)

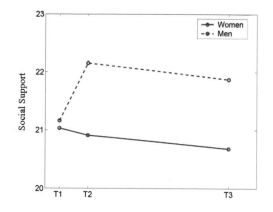

*Figure 8. Mean Level Changes in Social Support by Gender*

Note. Higher values indicate more social support (Range 5 – 25)

*Cut-off values*

For practical purposes, Zigmond and Snaith (1983) recommended three cut-off scores for the anxiety subscale of the HADS: 0-7 was seen as normal, 8-10 as borderline and $\geq 11$ as the optimal cut-off score for anxiety disorders. Table 22 compares the percentages of men and women in the different categories for depressive and anxiety disorders. In the present study, women consistently reported more anxiety symptoms across all measurement points. However, the most marked difference in anxiety occurred before surgery, with roughly 41% of women reporting anxiety at least with a borderline value indicative of an anxiety syndrome (men: 27.3%). For major depression, the recommended cut-off value of the PHQ is $\geq 10$, including the specific items that are indispensable for the diagnosis of major depression. Before CABG surgery, 12.1% of women versus 5.9% of men had a PHQ score indicative of major depression ($p < 0.05$). At the second and third measurement points this gender difference diminished.

**Table 22. Gender Differences in Percentages of Low versus High Anxiety and Depression: Significance of $\chi^2$-test**

|  | Men n= 289 | Women n= 66 | $\chi^2$ | df | p | p |
|---|---|---|---|---|---|---|
| Anxiety T1 High % | 27.3 | 40.9 | 4.65 | 1 | 0.03 | * |
| Depression T1 High % | 5.9 | 12.1 | 3.2 | 1 | 0.07 | + |
| Anxiety T2 High % | 15.2 | 24.2 | 3.11 | 1 | 0.08 | + |
| Depression T2 High % | 5.5 | 9.1 | 1.17 | 1 | 0.28 | n.s. |
| Anxiety T3 High % | 19.0 | 28.8 | 3.05 | 1 | 0.08 | + |
| DepressionT3 High % | 5.9 | 9.1 | 0.91 | 1 | 0.34 | n.s. |

Notes. n.s. non significant $+p < 0.10$ $*p < 0.05$

## Postoperative Physical Functioning

At all time points, patients were asked to rate their physical functioning on a three-point scale and the degree to which they currently felt impaired by their health status on a two-point scale. Means and standard deviations for the study variables are presented in Table 23.

**Table 23. Means and Standard Deviations for Physical Functioning by Gender**

| Physical functioning | Men n= 289 | | Women n= 66 | |
|---|---|---|---|---|
|  | M | SD | M | SD |
| T1 | 56.06 | 26.00 | 46.74 | 24.39 |
| T2 | 63.32 | 25.09 | 52.05 | 22.45 |
| T3 | 69.10 | 27.17 | 57.95 | 25.28 |

Note. Range from 0 to 100, higher values indicating better physical functioning

Figure 9 shows the development of physical functioning over time for men and women. Using SPSS GLM REPEATED MEASURES, a 2 (gender) by 3 (measurement points) repeated measures analysis of variance (ANOVA) yielded significant changes in physical functioning across all measurement points ($F(2,351) = 24,96$, $p < 0.01$: $Eta^2 = 0.12$). Because the Mauchly test indicated a significant departure from sphericity (i.e. from homogeneity of variances of pairwise differences between variables), and in response to the slight departures from assumptions underlying repeated measures ANOVAs, the conservative Greenhouse-Geisser correction to the tests of significance was applied. The effect remained significant (critical value for an alpha level of 0.05: $F_{corrected}(1.187,662.88) = 27,76$). Pairwise comparisons demonstrated significant changes from T1 to T2 ($p < 0.01$) and from T2 to T3 ($p < 0.01$). With regard to gender, the analysis of the between-subjects factor (gender) also revealed a major effect ($F(1,353) = 12,72$, $p < 0.01$: $Eta^2 = 0.04$), whereas men and women did not differ in the course of their physiological recovery over time.

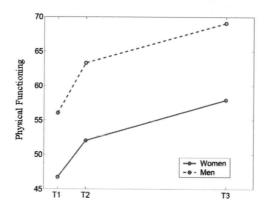

**Figure 9. Mean Level Changes in Physical Functioning by Gender**

Note. Higher values indicate better physical functioning (Range 0-100)

*Do more women than men experience a deterioration of their physical functioning (PF)?* This question was addressed by creating three groups – a PF-gain group, a PF-loss group and a PF-stable group – following the procedure suggested by Mallik et al. (2005). For each group, the measure at baseline was subtracted from the equivalent measure at follow-up 2 months later and 1 year later, respectively. For each wave (T1-T2; T2-T3), these scores were used to create three change groups. The patient's physical functioning was considered improved (gain group) or deteriorated (loss group), if the score changed more than 5 points in either direction at T2 or T3, respectively. It was expected that more women than men experienced a deterioration in physical functioning at T2.

Repeated measures ANOVAs at the beginning of this section demonstrated a trend towards improvement of physical functioning. However, surgery was not successful for *all* patients. Two months after surgery, physical functioning had improved in 53.2% of patients (54% men, 50% women). 14.4% of patients had no change (14.2% men, 15.2% women) and in 32.4% (31.8% men, 34.8% women) of the patients the physical functioning was worse than prior to surgery. However, the gender differences in the gain and loss groups did not reach significance. Changes after 1 year compared to the status 2 months after surgery were positive for 56.3% of the patients, stayed the same for 14.1% and worsened for 29.6%. Again, in contrast to the expectations, *gender* differences in changes were not significant.

Men's and women's health status improved 2 months after surgery compared to the status prior to surgery, even though they differed in physical functioning, depression and anxiety before surgery. The degree of improvement over time was similar in both genders and continued over the first postoperative year. An increase in physical functioning corresponded to a decrease in depression and anxiety after surgery. However, almost one third of the patients did not experience an improvement in physical functioning 2 months after surgery. Men and women did not differ in their reporting of social support before surgery. However, 2 months after surgery, men were receiving more support than women.

### 4.2.2 Stress Factors after Surgery

This section deals with patients' perceived stress through housework, their social support and the multiple associations with depression and physical functioning. First, men and women are compared in the categories of the Household Questionnaire. Second, relationships with outcome variables are outlined.

**Domestic Work**

More women than men reported that they generally perform household tasks (Table 24). This difference, however, was only of marginal significance ($p < 0.08$). A significant difference emerged when patients were asked how many *hours* they spent per day on these activities. The analysis was performed with a dichotomous variable indicating time spent on housework of less than 3 hours and more than 3 hours. Many more women than men reported spending more than 3 hours per day. Additionally, patients were asked who supported them in their household chores. Multiple answers were permitted. Whereas more men than women reported support by a partner, more women than men reported support by their children. Roughly 20% of women had no support at all in these activities in contrast to 7% of men (p < 0.01).

**Table 24. Gender Differences in Housework: $\chi^2$-tests**

| Variables | Men n= 289 | Women n= 66 | $\chi^2$ | df | p | |
|---|---|---|---|---|---|---|
| Do you perform housework? | 73.0 | 83.3 | 3.05 | 1 | 0.08 | + |
| How many hours? | | | 27.51 | 3 | 0.001 | ** |
| <3 h/day | 86.5 | 59.1 | 5.71 | 1 | 0.017 | * |
| >3 h/day | 13.5 | 40.9 | 26.68 | 1 | 0.001 | ** |
| Support by partner[a] | 66.1 | 45.5 | 9.736 | 1 | 0.002 | ** |
| Support by children | 15.6 | 39.4 | 19.06 | 1 | 0.001 | ** |
| Support by someone else | 7.3 | 10.6 | 0.82 | 1 | 0.36 | n.s. |
| No support | 6.9 | 19.7 | 10.37 | 1 | 0.001 | ** |
| High stress through housework | 18.3 | 36.4 | 10.28 | 1 | 0.001 | ** |

Notes. +p < 0.10 *p < 0.05 **p < 0.01

Multiple answers were permitted with respect to support

Women not only spent more time on housework, they also felt more stressed by these activities. Twice as many women as men reported that they felt rather or very stressed by their housework.

### Relationships between Housework and Wellbeing

The question is whether women engage too much in household activities in an early stage of recovery and therefore perform less well in terms of psychological and physiological adaptation. In order to answer this question, planned correlations were first inspected including age, partner status and risk scores. Second, the influence of engagement in household tasks on depression and physical functioning was examined.

Table 25 shows planned Pearson's correlations between household tasks, depression, physical functioning and the various characteristics mentioned above. The analyses demonstrate that the time spent on housework was independent of most of the other parameters except for a weak positive association between time spent on housework and the stress caused by it and time and age in men. The relationships between *time* spent on housework and physical functioning or depression, respectively, were, in contrast to the assumptions, close to zero. However, housework stress was significantly associated with depression and physical functioning in both men and women: individuals reporting more stress through household tasks tended to be more depressive and displayed lower physical functioning than individuals with less stress. While social support was significantly associated with depression and physical functioning in men, this was only true for depression in women. This observation holds, when not only the significance of correlations is taken into account, but also the effect size of coefficients. In women, the correlation between social support and physical functioning was close to zero at both measurement points (r = 0.03 / r = 0.04). Furthermore, social support was associated with depression in both genders, whereas the association of social support and housework stress was only significant in women. Because the overall relationships between depression and housework stress were small to moderate in both genders, both constructs are presumably largely independent.

**Table 25. Relationships between Housework, Social Support, Personal Characteristics, Physical Functioning and Depression: Pearson's Correlations at T2 and T3 (Men above Diagonal)**

| | | Men n = 289 | | | | | | | | | | |
|---|---|---|---|---|---|---|---|---|---|---|---|---|
| | | 1 | 2 | 3 | 4 | 5 | 6 | 7 | 8 | 9 | 10 | 11 |
| Women n= 66 | 1 Age | | 0.07 | 0.02 | 0.06 | 0.15** | -0.05 | 0.10 | -0.25** | -0.06 | -0.17** | -0.08 |
| | 2 Partner Status | 0.31* (3) | | -0.08 | 0.03 | 0.10(4) | 0.13**(4) | -0.32** | -0.22** | 0.15** | -0.20** | 0.18** |
| | 3 Fram. Score (1) | 0.16 | 0.08 | | 0.06 | -0.02 | 0.10 | -0.00 | -0.14* | 0.12 | -0.17** | 0.13* |
| | 4 EuroSCORE (1) | 0.03 | 0.10 | -0.16 | | 0.03 | 0.04 | -0.04 | -0.09 | 0.09 | -0.18** | 0.13* |
| | 5 Household Time T2 | 0.11 | -0.13(4) | -0.05 | 0.03 | | 0.21**(4) | -0.08 | -0.03 | 0.00 | -0.04 | -0.02 |
| | 6 Housework stress T2 | -0.08 | -0.03(4) | -0.07 | -0.01 | 0.08(4) | | -0.11 | -0.33** | 0.35** | -0.34** | 0.29** |
| | 7 Social Support T2 | -0.02 | -0.30* | 0.10 | 0.02 | 0.09 | -0.31* | | 0.13* | -0.23** | 0.16** | -0.23** |
| | 8 PF T2 | -0.29* | -0.14 | -0.04 | -0.13 | 0.14 | -0.26* | -0.03 | | -0.54** | 0.71** | -0.46** |
| | 9 Depression T2 (2) | 0.01 | -0.05(3) | 0.06 | -0.02 | 0.04 | 0.30** | -0.35** | -0.23 | | -0.46** | 0.66** |
| | 10 PF T3 | -0.18 | -0.11 | -0.09 | -0.11 | 0.12 | -0.18 | -0.04 | 0.60** | -0.27 | | -0.60** |
| | 11 Depression T3 (2) | -0.19 | -0.07 | 0.14 | -0.06 | -0.04 | 0.18 | -0.26* | -0.16(3) | 0.67** | -0.37** | |

Notes. +p < 0.10 *p < 0.05 **p < 0.01

(1) Age excluded

(2) Square root transformation

(3) Grey cells: All correlations between person characteristics and physical functioning and depression, respectively, were tested for gender differences. Marginal gender difference:

a) age –partner status (p < 0.10)

b) depression – partner status (p < 0.10)

Significant gender difference: c) depression – physical functioning (p < 0.01)

(4) φ-correlations for categorical data

To examine the influence of household activities on depression and physical functioning, sequential (hierarchical) multiple regression analyses were conducted using SPSS REGRESSION. The first two analyses were cross-sectional at T2, with depression and physical functioning as outcome variables (Table 26 and Table 27). Age, partner status and risk scores were considered as rival predictors and were thus included as control variables in the first step, whereas time and stress were included in the second and third step, respectively. The third and fourth analyses were conducted to demonstrate potential effects of household activities on the *change* in depression and physical functioning from the second to the third measurement point. To assess the change in depression and physical functioning, the respective baseline score – depression or physical functioning at T2 – was included in the equation in the first step. The rival predictors were included in the second step, time and stress in the third or fourth step, respectively. Table 26 shows the results of the cross-sectional regression analyses for men and women separately with $R^2$ displaying the percentage of variance explained and $\Delta R^2$ reflecting the change in variance (after adding the control variables, housework stress, social support and time on household). The coefficient $\beta$ specifies the regression weights.

**Table 26. Sequential (Hierarchical) Multiple Regression of Depression on Housework**

| Depression T2[2] | Men n= 289 | | | Women n= 66 | | |
|---|---|---|---|---|---|---|
| | $R^2$ | $\Delta R^2$ | $\beta$ | $R^2$ | $\Delta R^2$ | $\beta$ |
| Model I: Control variables [1] | 0.05 | 0.05** | | 0.01 | 0.01 | |
| Model II: Social support added | 0.08 | 0.03** | -0.18** | 0.17 | 0.16** | -0.36** |
| Model III: Time on household added | 0.08 | 0.00 | -0.08 | 0.17 | 0.00 | 0.04 |
| Model IV: Housework stress added | 0.18 | 0.10** | 0.33** | 0.20 | 0.03 | 0.19 |

Notes. +p < 0.10 *p < 0.05 **p < 0.01

(1) Age, partner status, risk scores

(2) Square root transformed variable

**Table 27. Sequential (Hierarchical) Multiple Regression of Physical Functioning on Housework**

| Physical functioning T2 | Men n= 289 | | | Women n= 66 | | |
|---|---|---|---|---|---|---|
| | $R^2$ | $\Delta R^2$ | $\beta$ | $R^2$ | $\Delta R^2$ | $\beta$ |
| Model I: Control variables [1] | 0.11 | 0.11** | | 0.09 | 0.09 | |
| Model II: Social support added | 0.12 | 0.01* | 0.10+ | 0.10 | 0.00 | -0.20 |
| Model III: Time on household added | 0.12 | 0.00 | 0.08 | 0.13 | 0.03 | 0.21 |
| Model IV: Housework stress added | 0.22 | 0.10** | -0.33** | 0.24 | 0.12** | -0.37** |

Notes. +p < 0.10 *p < 0.05 **p < 0.01

(1) Age, partner status, risk scores

After controlling for age, partner status and clinical risk factors, low social support still significantly contributed to higher depression levels in both genders (Table 26). Only in men, stress through housework was associated with higher levels of depression. With regard to physical functioning, social support was only marginally significant after adjusting for control variables, whereas stress through housework had a significant impact in both genders. The *time* spent on housework was not associated with depression or physical functioning in either men or women. In the second set of analyses, neither social support nor time spent on housework had an influence on the *change* in depression (from T2 to T3) or *change* in physical functioning (from T2 to T3). Additionally, in women the housework stress did not contribute to the change in depression and physical functioning over time ($\beta$ = -0.05, n.s.) whereas in men housework stress contributed significantly to the change in physical functioning ($\beta$ = -0.13, p < 0.01). This effect still remained significant ($\beta$ = -0.12, p < 0.01), if depression at the second measurement point was controlled for. In other words, men who felt stressed by housework 2 months after surgery experienced a change to the worse in physical functioning over time.

In summary, 6 to 8 weeks after surgery, women worked more hours at home than men. Twice as many women as men expressed feelings of stress caused by housework. In both men and women, cross-sectionally the stress through housework was associated with physical functioning and depression. In contrast, the *time* that both men and women spent on housework did not have an effect on either depression or physical functioning. Surprisingly, the data showed that in men, not in women, stress through housework led to a deterioration in physical functioning over time after adjustment for health status, age, partner status and social support.

## 4.3   Predictive Relationship between Physical Functioning and Depression

In the final section the results of the analyses are condensed into the concise pattern of an analytic path model. Here, two questions were in the centre of interest: (1) *Do patients who display more depressive symptoms preoperatively or 2 months after surgery experience lower levels of physical functioning at later time points?* The direction of influence is not clear and has been controversial, since the alternative predictive direction – an effect of physical functioning on depression – is also plausible. Patients who experience physical limitations could react with depression over time. This topic relates to causal relationships and can only be answered by analyses with longitudinal data. The second question concerns gender differences within the model. (2) *Do men and women differ with regard to the proposed paths?*

In order to answer these questions, a path model was created. Using AMOS Structural Equation Modeling, cross-sectional and prospective relationships of depression and physical functioning were tested by a cross-lagged panel design. In such a design three relationships have to be included in the model to allow for inference of predictive direction: (a) longitudinal correlations among the three depression measures and the three measures of physical functioning; (b) cross-sectional correlations between depression and physical functioning; (c) the cross-lagged correlations between depression and physical functioning. Only if the respective predictor (depression or physical functioning) made an independent contribution to the criterion (physical functioning and depression) after controlling for the effects at earlier time points and cross-sectional associations would a causal interpretation be justified. Figure 10 shows the possible cross-lagged paths.

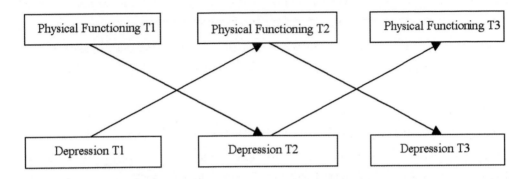

*Figure 10. The Proposed Structural Equation Model:*
*Relationships between Physical Functioning and Depression over Time*

Structural Equation Modeling allows the estimation of underlying latent information. In order to use this utility, depression and physical functioning were understood as latent constructs in this process. At all three measurement points, the latent constructs were estimated by two randomly selected split-half "subtests" (Arbuckle and Wollke, 1995; see Vauth et al., 2007). The conventional $\chi^2$-test can be distorted by larger sample sizes, which was the case in the present study ($\chi^2 = 139.8$, df $= 39$, p $< 0.01$). However, additional indices that are robust to sample size showed acceptable fit indices: overall fit: CMIN/df $= 3.584$; RMSEA $= 0.067$; CFI $= 0.98$; NFI $= 0.97$. The structural model was also fitted with male data and female data separately and yielded similar results to those reported above. The reliability and validity of the measurement model was good. All indicators could be considered to represent attributes of the corresponding constructs physical functioning and depression. Indicator reliability was ranging from 0.85 to 0.98. Multiple model-data-fit indices were used to assess the degree to which the structural model fitted the data.

Figure 11 presents the standardized estimates for the structural model specifying the causal relationships between depression and physical functioning. The stability effects of both variables were assessed through the unidirectional paths linking the same latent variable from the earlier measurement points to the later measurement points. As expected, the best predictors for depression at the second and third measurement point were the depression scores at earlier time points (i.e. the baseline scores at T1 and T2, respectively). The stability effects were lower from the first to the second measurement point than from the second to the third measurement point. With regard to cross-sectional associations, a low level of physical functioning was associated with higher depression rates at all time points.

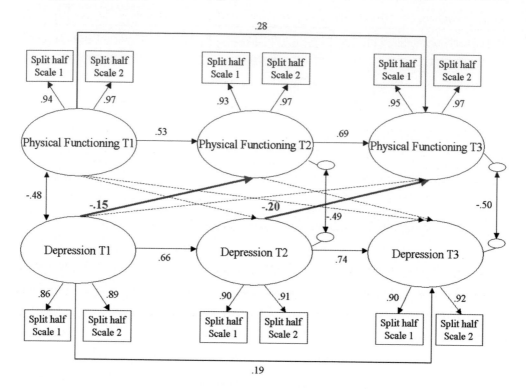

***Figure 11. Realized Cross-lagged Panel Model:***
***Testing the Relationship between Physical Functioning and Depression over Time.***

Notes. Rectangles indicate observed indicator variables. Ovals indicate unobserved latent variables.

Numbers at headed arrows indicate standardized regression weights.

All paths shown are significant at $p < 0.05$ except for those drawn with a broken line.

All parameters in this model were unconstrained.

The cross-lagged unidirectional paths between depression and physical functioning specified the predictive contributions of depression at previous measurement points to physical functioning at later measurement points as well as the predictive contribution of physical functioning at previous measurement points to changes in depression at later time points. The paths from prior physical functioning to later depression were not significant. In contrast, prior depression did significantly relate to later physical functioning. This means that depression showed predictive priority over physical functioning, and this predictive priority could be demonstrated for both time intervals.

Within a multi-group model comparison it was tested whether gender differences were present in the predictive relationships between depression and physical functioning. The multi-group analysis is an efficient statistical test to confirm moderator effects such as gender by estimating causal effects for men and women simultaneously. To do so, constraints were used that required the cross-lagged regression weights to be equal in men and women. This constrained model did not differ significantly from the unconstrained model described above ($\chi^2_{diff}$ = 2.773, p = 0.60). This means that the cross-lagged regression weights – the longitudinal correlations between depression and physical functioning – did not differ between men and women. Thus, the alternative hypothesis that the pattern of relationships of depression and physical functioning in men differs significantly from that in women must be rejected. Subsequently, the model based on the entire sample was used to answer the first question concerning the causal influence of physical functioning and depression.

After controlling for the respective cross-sectional and baseline scores, depression showed a pronounced predictive priority over physical functioning. This means that higher depression scores led to worse physical functioning at later time points and not vice versa. Men and women did not differ with respect to the pattern of these relationships: the model described above was valid for both genders.

# 5 DISCUSSION

There are three key results that will be discussed. First, in section 4.1, depression emerged as the most important psychosocial risk factor for both mortality and physical functioning in the entire sample, while education mediated the relationship between gender and mortality. The predictive priority of depression over physical functioning was confirmed in a cross-lagged panel design, in which cross-sectional associations and baseline scores were controlled for. Second, section 4.2 showed comparable improvement for both men and women after surgery concerning the mean scores of physical functioning and depression. Third, strain through housework in the early phase of recovery proved to be associated negatively with physical functioning and positively with depression in both men and women. These three results will now be discussed with regard to the baseline health status. In addition, methodological considerations, limitations of the study and clinical implications will be outlined.

## 5.1 Gender Differences in Outcome

In the present study, the all-cause mortality rate of women after CABG surgery appeared to be twice that of men. For the analysis, a time period of 1 year after surgery had been selected. The majority of studies (e.g. Vaccarino et al., 2002, Regitz-Zagrosek et al., 2004) also found gender differences in early mortality, which is defined as mortality within 28 days after surgery. Only a few studies went beyond this short term. If a survival time of over 1 year was considered, either no gender differences were found or female gender was even shown to be a predictor for an improved survival rate (Brandrup-Wognsen et al., 1996; Toumpoulis et al., 2006). In contrast, the gender ratio of the present analysis with regard to the survival rate equalled that of the results for early mortality.

Previous studies in search of an explanation of these gender differences have yielded quite diverse results. In some studies, after adjustment for clinical risk factors, the gender differences in early mortality disappeared (Abramov et al., 2000; Toumpoulis et al., 2006). In other studies (e.g. Regitz-Zagrosek et al., 2004; Vaccarino et al., 2002), the gender gap remained visible. Most of these studies, however, were only retrospective, which implies that psychosocial risk factors could not enter adequately into the analysis. In contrast to these earlier studies, the present study was designed as prospective, thus allowing a rich variety of socioeconomic, clinical and psychosocial risk factors to be included. By this construction, the relative importance of psychosocial factors in comparison with the classical clinical risk factors, which have been more closely examined in earlier analyses, could be demonstrated.

Two main groups of hypotheses were tested to explain the gender difference in mortality after CABG. The first group examined the moderator status of gender, while the second concerned the mediator status of risk factors. The first group refers to the fact that risk factors have a stronger impact on wellbeing in women than in men, which is usually indicated by interactions. The second type of hypothesis alludes to the fact that some risk factors appear predominantly in women. If these risk factors are, in turn, similarly related to mortality in men and in women, they can explain the gender difference in mortality and physical functioning. Three different types of potential mediator or moderator variables – clinical risk factors, sociodemographic variables and psychosocial variables – provide the framework for the following presentation.

### 5.1.1 Clinical Risk Factors

On this topic a large variety of literature is available. However, only few studies dealt with the interaction of clinical and psychosocial variables. In the present thesis gender differences in clinical factors are discussed only briefly, to assess the impact of psychosocial factors, which will be looked at in more detail.

As shown in section 5.1, there was a trend that women displayed more risk factors than men. More women had a history of hypertension, congestive heart failure and neurological complications after surgery, whereas men were more likely to be smokers. LVEF was found to be similar in men and women. These findings are congruent with the results of Vaccarino et al. (2003) who prospectively studied gender differences in bypass patients. However, with respect to diabetes, the gender difference in the present study did not reach significance, although the rates were comparable to those in Vaccarino's study in terms of absolute numbers.

In order to summarize the risk factors, two scores were calculated: the Framingham Score and the EuroSCORE. The Framingham Score was originally constructed for the purpose of predicting the risk of myocardial infarction (Wilson et al., 1998), which was not the goal of the present study. Rather the score was used here to include the "classical" risk factors such as diabetes and smoking. Evidently, this risk score did not contribute to the prediction of either mortality or physical functioning in this population, in which the event had already occurred. In contrast, the EuroSCORE, which was designed to predict the mortality risk after bypass surgery (Nashef et al., 1999), did contribute significantly. In fact, it was the dominant predictor for mortality. However, the EuroSCORE alone did not explain the marked gender difference in mortality. A possible source of this lack may lie in the special role of age with respect to gender.

On the basis of this conjecture age was deliberately excluded from the calculation of the EuroSCORE. As will be shown in section 5.1.2, age did mediate relationship between gender and mortality – a result that could not be inferred from the EuroSCORE.

Apart from mortality as an objective outcome parameter, it was essential to examine the subjective health status. Risk factors for low physical functioning and mortality only partly coincided. Clinical risk factors for low physical functioning were renal failure, heart failure und a high body mass index. All these risk factors are chronic conditions and therefore it seems no surprise that they affect the quality of life and physical functioning. For example, heart failure diminishes the quality of life in several ways: the patients easily fatigue, experience breathlessness, and have swollen ankles (Kaltenbach and Olbrich, 2000). In contrast to the expectations, clinical risk factors were not more strongly related to either mortality or physical functioning in women. However, a trend in the expected direction was observed for LVEF, hypertension, hyperlipidemia and incomplete revascularization and deserves attention in studies with larger samples.

Another result that warrants attention is that the rate of incomplete revascularization was higher in women, a fact that was also associated with their higher mortality. Only few studies have directly or indirectly addressed this issue. Osswald et al. (2001) stated that the lower number of bypass grafts and the lower use of arterial grafts in women compared with men (for the same extent of CHD) suggested incomplete revascularization and would be likely to have an impact on long-term mortality. Other studies (Humphries et al., 2007; Blankstein et al., 2005) pointed out that after adjustment for body surface area (BSA) the gender difference diminished. As BSA is considered a surrogate for vessel size it is likely that patients with low BSA are at higher risk because small coronary arteries might be more difficult to operate upon. However, the relationship between gender, BSA and vessel size is complex. To calculate the ratio of diseased vessels to grafted vessels might be an effective way of estimating the individual risk. Incomplete revascularization as defined by the calculation of this ratio showed an only weak relationship with mortality but may be of some clinical importance, and deserves additional study.

## 5.1.2 Sociodemographic Risk Factors

The present study is characterized by the fact that its women were older than men at the time of operation, had a lower education level and were more likely to live alone. These findings are in accordance with those of previous investigations (Vaccarino et al., 2003; Bute et al., 2003; Ai et al., 1997; Moore, 1995). Up to now, only few studies on CABG have included both socioeconomic and psychosocial variables.

Women in this study were, on average, 69 years old and thus approximately 5 years older than men. This is in accordance with the population of bypass patients in a recent study by Vaccarino et al. (2003). In contrast, Mitchell et al. (2005) pointed out that with respect to age the previously usual 10-year gap has decreased over the past few years, and is now even vanishing. However, not only was the entire patient population in the present study on average older than the sample of Mitchell et al., but the female patients were also older than the males. This fact may point to a more complex history in women and has to be taken into account in the interpretation of the results. Age, as a risk factor for mortality mediated the relationship between gender and mortality, which means that adjustment for age appeared to diminish the gender gap in this regard.

**Partner Status and Social Support**

Although relatively more women than men were living alone, they did not report less emotional support before the operation. Neither social support at this time point nor partner status was associated with mortality. Moreover, only in men was there a relationship between social support and physical functioning, which appeared to be rather weak. How can the results of this study be explained in view of previous findings, which advocated the view that a lack of social support lengthens the hospitalization of male CHD patients (Kulik and Mahler, 1989), accelerates the progression of CHD and even leads to premature death (Zöller, 1999)?

In this context, there are some possible explanations for the lacking association between partner status, social support and mortality. The data show that shortly before surgery most patients reported a high degree of social support. In times of adverse life events there is a need for social support and there are normative expectations for its provision, both on the part of the patient and on the part of the partner. At such times, lack of support is unlikely and would be most consequential (Elizur and Hirsh, 1999). It is also not surprising that most patients, undergoing a difficult surgery, turn to their spouses or children and, as a consequence, report high levels of emotional support. This leads – from a statistical perspective – to a lack of variance and consequently to an underestimation of associations. The failure to identify a relationship between emotional support and mortality or physical functioning is in line with the findings of Barry et al. (2006) and Elizur and Hirsh (1999), who also studied various aspects of social support in bypass patients. These authors detected a correlation between instrumental support and mental health status on the one hand (Barry et al., 2006) and marital satisfaction and physical functioning on the other hand (Elizur and Hirsh, 1999). This leads to the assumption that one reason for the lacking association between social support and mortality (or the weak correlation between social support and physical functioning) may lie within the construct itself. Generally, a distinction can be made between emotional and instrumental support, as well as distinguishing between qualitative and quantitative aspects. Given the low variance of emotional support in this study, other components may be more valid in the context of an upcoming operation and should be added to future studies.

**Socioeconomic Status**

Socioeconomic status (SES) is a construct manifesting itself through a variety of indicators. Here, education level was selected as a valid indicator for SES. In this study fewer women than men had vocational training. In women, the education level was correlated with mortality, in the entire sample also with physical functioning. As shown in section 4.1, it mediated the relationship between gender and mortality, thus partly explaining the gender gap in mortality. This result cannot easily be compared with that of other studies, since the data situation with respect to gender differences after CABG is poor. However, some studies have shown that men and women with a low education level have a higher risk of dying of CHD (Albus and Siegrist, 2005). Lacey and Walters (2003) found that women with lower SES showed poorer recovery after MI than men. One reason for this finding may be that a low education level is often related to adverse health behaviour, which, in turn, is associated with a less favourable profile of clinical risk factors (Albus & Siegrist, 2005). For both men and women, low socioeconomic status is associated with lifestyle behaviours that increase one's susceptibility to cardiac disease: heavy smoking, increased stress, unhealthy eating habits, and physical inactivity (Brezinka and Kittel, 1996). Wamala et al. (2000) reported that women in unskilled positions were at a far greater risk of developing CHD than academic women. There is some evidence that domestic roles are less flexible in working class homes (Lacey and Walters, 2005). Moreover, lack of access to a car can be important in terms of physical limitations. This is in line with findings from another study showing that for women restricted mobility was one of the most important reasons not to attend rehabilitation programmes (Grande, 2002). From a more general point of view, Sieverding (1995) indicated that paid work and career building have a number of positive effects that can protect against harmful factors, including, most notably, economic and social independence as well as greater social support.

If measured through education level, SES is a risk factor which, to a great extent, can be assumed to be largely dependent on cohort effects. Many women of the present patient cohort might not have had the chance of vocational training or access to higher education. Therefore, the ratio of men and women in whom a low SES affects mortality and physical functioning is likely to change in the future. The exact paths of education level exerting its influence on mortality and its interaction with stress related to surgery should be assessed in future studies. Moreover, the consequences of societal changes and demands need to be continually documented.

From the point of view of Hobfoll and Wells (1998) health, socio-economic status and partnership can be regarded as resources. As part of his theory of "conservation of resources" Hobfoll states that a loss of resources is the main source of stress. If only few resources are available, any loss causes severe damage, while gaining new resources is harder to achieve. This insight certainly applies to the situation before and after CABG surgery. On average, women had initially fewer resources than men. Thus, a vicious cycle is more likely to emerge, with the individual becoming more and more susceptible and being hampered in effectively coping with problems. Such "loss spirals" are particularly dangerous for individuals who lack economic and social support and psychological resources (Hobfoll and Schumm, 2004). In the perioperative setting of CABG, such a lack of resources may lead to stressful experiences. Since poverty places individuals at the limit of their resources in many domains, an additional stress factor like surgery may be disastrous, because there are limited resources to be mobilized. The close dependencies described may well serve as a theoretical explanatory framework for the relationship between socio-economic status and mortality in women as presented here.

### 5.1.3 Preoperative Depression and Anxiety

Before surgery, anxiety scores of more than 40% in the group of women and 30% in the group of men were within a range indicative of at least moderate symptoms of an anxiety disorder. At the same time, women had considerably higher average levels of depression than men. They were twice as likely as men to be in a range indicative of major depression. This ratio with regard to depression is similar to those reported in epidemiological studies of psychiatric disorders in the general community (Weissman et al., 1996). The reasons for the higher depression rates remain controversial. Some authors have suggested that it may be more socially accepted for women to report depressive symptoms than it is for men (Davison and Neale, 2002), while others have speculated that in times of stress women have a stronger tendency toward "ruminating" around the stressor and are therefore more likely to develop depression (Nolen-Hoeksema, 2001).

The model that fitted the data best in the entire sample contained depression as a risk factor next to age and the EuroSCORE. Previous studies have shown that depression is an independent risk factor for mortality after MI (Frasure-Smith et al., 1999), congestive heart failure (Jiang et al., 2001) and CHD (Barefoot et al., 1996). However, only few studies have investigated whether depression affects long-term outcomes in CABG patients. Some of these studies have been limited by their lack of statistical power (e.g. Connerney et al., 2001) and therefore could not prove the effect of depression on mortality. Furthermore, the small sample sizes did not allow the adjustment of risk factors. Yet, the results of the present study are consistent with the data of a large prospective study by Blumenthal et al. (2003), who found an association between depression and mortality in patients who had been followed-up for up to 12 years.

It was hypothesized that the higher depression rates in women, on the one hand, and the relationship between depression and mortality, on the other hand, would partly explain the gender difference in mortality. However, only a small proportion of the gender difference in mortality could be explained by different prevalence rates of depression in men versus women. This is not surprising given the relatively low correlation between depression and mortality and may explain that depression does not account for a great proportion of the variance with respect to mortality. Further research should focus on clarifying the relationship between depression and mortality. Ideally, the depression variable should be split up into distinct parts – one part bearing a strong relationship with mortality and a second category that contains the portion of variance in the depression variable that is irrelevant for the prediction of mortality. Both predictions and interventions could then focus on the most pertinent facets of depression, surpassing the uncertainties surrounding low correlations.

Indeed the results of this study already hint at more specific relations. Before surgery, depression was closely associated with anxiety, the association being even more marked in women. Anxiety itself did not predict mortality and did not remain significant as a predictor for physical functioning after adjustment for other psychosocial risk factors. There is a clear overlap of anxiety and depression and a decrease in both parameters postoperatively. Consequently, one may assume that some depressive symptoms are associated with anxiety before surgery; these facets of depression may disappear post-operatively, thereby having no further impact on mortality.

Further research should illuminate which aspects of depression are the best predictors for deterioration of the patient's health status. In this regard, mortality is only the utmost criterion, failing to grasp the full variance of health developments. The consideration of health-related quality of life might thus yield an enriched picture of the pertinent relations and be an indispensable source for further analyses. In this study, physical functioning as a subjective outcome parameter indicated the physical component of subjective health-related quality of life.

Some of the relationships between depression and physical functioning are discussed in the following sections.

## 5.2 Gender Aspects in Recovery

This section deals with the recovery process after surgery. Here, the influence of daily chores on physical functioning as well as the development of depression and physical functioning over time are taken into account.

### 5.2.1 Domestic Work

One of the hypotheses in section 2.1 was that women would resume daily chores shortly after surgery and would therefore spend more time on household chores than men. Stress caused by household activities should therefore be higher for women than for men and impair physical functioning and increase depression. In fact, the results showed that already a few weeks after surgery women spent much more time on daily chores than men. In accordance with the time spent on household chores, twice as many women as men reported being highly stressed by their chores.

There is some evidence from other studies to show that the recovery after a heart attack or a bypass surgery with respect to the resumption of household activities differs considerably between men and women. Rose et al. (1996) showed that female patients, soon after a heart attack, worked more hours in the household than their husbands, whereas in contrast, male patients experienced a significant relief by their spouses from household duties in the weeks after their heart attack. The results of Artinian and Duggan (1995) and King et al. (1994) show that women feel more strongly restricted by their household chores than men. Whereas Rose et al. (1996) asked patients to report the type and amount of activities, Artinian and Duggan together with King et al. assessed the subjective stress on a continuous scale. Despite the variation of measurements, the results are in line with those of the present study and can be explained by two factors. First, women typically take on more household responsibilities than men. Thus, it is not surprising that they feel more stressed due to household chores. Second, women generally have fewer available resources than men. They live more frequently alone and receive less social support. Accordingly, several authors (Jenson et al., 2003; Lemos et al., 2003) assume that women's working in the household soon after the operation is an important risk factor. Jenson et al. (2003) demonstrated that activities of women are, unlike those of men, not distributed over the whole day, but are condensed within a shorter period of time. Therefore Jenson et al. assume that a premature resumption of household activities, in their condensed mode, could be particularly damaging for women. In a similar way, the present study revealed no relationship between the *time* men or women spent on household activities on the one hand and physical functioning or depression on the other hand. In fact, the only trend observed was a *positive* relationship between time spent on housework and ratings of physical functioning in women. It seems likely that the amount of time in this context rather reflects a better health status. When focusing on perceived stress due to housework, a different picture appears. This source of stress was cross-sectionally associated with depression and reduced physical functioning in both genders. Surprisingly, the data showed that in men, but not in women, stress due to housework predicted deterioration in physical functioning over time, after adjustment for depression, health status, sociodemographic variables and social support. This allows for various interpretations. One could assume that women receive less support than men because they are more often living alone or, if living with a partner, feel pressured to resume their daily chores as soon as possible. However, for some women of this age cohort, working in the house may be part of their personal identity (Boogard and Broidy, 1985), i.e. a stabilizing factor reinforcing that, despite their illness they are still the person they used to be. This positive stabilizing factor may outweigh the negative impact of physical exertion that housework brings about. By contrast, men generally feel less responsible for the household. Therefore, men after surgery seem to experience household tasks as stressful even when spending comparatively little time with it. In any case, the level of experienced stress is a predictor for an impaired sense of quality of life in men.

The fact that stress due to housework predicted a greater impairment in physical functioning in men compared to women can not yet be satisfactorily explained. Presently, there is only sparse data on this issue. In fact, validated instruments for the assessment of household chores still need to be developed. Moreover, the assignment of objective measurements beyond self-reports would be desirable. In addition, any such results may partly depend on experiences of a specific age cohort. Of course, changes in gender effects may be expected in the future, reflecting changes in traditional gender roles.

### 5.2.2   Changes in Physical Functioning and Depression

From research with healthy cohorts it has been established that women generally rate their subjective health status in terms of physical functioning as worse than men (Bullinger, 1995). This was true for the present sample of CABG patients as well: perioperatively women reported poorer physical functioning than men. However, before surgery, the gender difference within the sample of the present study was considerably more marked than in the age-comparable German norm. This gender difference could not be explained by either clinical or psychosocial risk factors only. Rather, all risk factors taken together provided an explanation of the gender difference in physical functioning. This means that after adjustment for clinical, socioeconomic and psychosocial risk factors the gender difference diminished considerably and gender only marginally contributed to the variance in physical functioning. The remaining contribution was approximately equivalent to the gender difference observed in the norm population. Possibly, being female is either associated with a stable tendency to report a worse health status or with greater attention paid to the own body (Nolen-Hoeksema, 2001). However, the same magnitude of gender difference in physical functioning as found in the present study is supported by previous findings (Emery et al., 2004; Mallik et al., 2005; Bute et al., 2003; Vaccarino et al., 2003).

The postoperative changes were considered by two different approaches: firstly the average changes in physical functioning were inspected. Here, men and women showed comparable average changes of physical functioning. That is to say that, in comparison to preoperative health status, both genders experienced a marked improvement in physical functioning over time. Secondly, it was assessed *how many* patients reported an improvement or worsening of their physical functioning and how these components related to each other. The *proportion* of patients who improved their physical functioning was more than 50%, whereas one third of patients experienced a decline in their condition of health. Both groups - those who rated their condition higher and those who rated it lower after the operation - consisted equally of men and women. Mallik et al. (2005) investigated the change over time in physical functioning and found that the proportion of women deteriorating after surgery was greater than that of men. Bute et al. (2003) and Vaccarino et al. (2003) found that, even after adjustment for baseline risk factors, women did not experience the same improvement in physical functioning as men did. In contrast, other studies (King, 2000; Sjoland et al., 1999) reported that, although men rated their quality of life pre-and postoperatively as better than women did, women showed a greater improvement in functional status postoperatively. No significant gender differences at all were found in a study by Hunt et al. (2000) on the subscale of physical functioning at the 1 year follow-up. However, the postoperative gender difference was 9 points and thus similar to that of our study. Therefore, this finding may reflect a lack of sufficient power ($n_{women} = 22$) rather than the absence of any gender differences. It can be concluded from the present results that women and men experience the same grade of improvement in terms of physical functioning, with the preoperative health status determining the future development.

As discussed in section 1.1.3 the rate of depression in women was double than that of men. The fact that the rate decreased among women but remained quite stable in men could be linked to two factors. First, women may react preoperatively with more depressive symptoms to the uncertainty and burden associated with the operation. Second, women in the present study had higher depression rates before surgery, but anxiety disorders were even more common: almost half of all women and a quarter of men experienced a set of symptoms which are at least within the range of clinically relevant anxiety disorders. In both genders these rates declined 2 months after surgery, but then remained generally stable. This is an indicator for the fact that the operation itself is a considerable stressor. This finding requires further research since it is known that (a) depression and anxiety overlap to a large extent, (b) anxiety may precede depression and may thus lead to depressive symptoms in the long term (Davison and Neale, 2002). To avoid from the start the development of depression in the group of bypass patients whose depression is assumed to be strongly associated with the situation, it seems important to detect anxiety disorders before patients fall into a vicious circle of anxiety and depression. In this respect, women may be more vulnerable, in that preoperative anxiety and depression were more strongly associated among women than among men (see section 1.1.3).

In summary, men and women experienced a comparable improvement in physical functioning and depression over time. By the fact that women in this study reported a worse quality of life after surgery, one can in no way conclude that they profited less from the operation than men. Both men and women experienced a substantial improvement in their quality of life. The fact that women rate their quality of life lower than men could partly be due to the perception of the situation and less to do with their actual condition of health. This question provides material for further research and, if need be, intervention.

## 5.3  Is Depression Predictive for Physical Functioning?

No other human organ is so closely associated with vitality and capability as the human heart. Therefore, it does not seem surprising that people suffering from CHD or undergoing a bypass operation see their vitality threatened, showing depressive symptoms in reaction to their illness and to the surgery. Changes in appetite, sleeping problems and a loss of energy are also symptoms of depression and suggest an overlap with physical symptoms. Surprisingly, the direction of predictive inference, as suggested in other studies (e.g. Faller et al., 1994), has not yet been clarified for this context: Does depression influence the quality of life after the operation or, vice versa, does the quality of life in terms of physical functioning lead to depressive symptoms?

So far, only unidirectional paths in the population of bypass patients have been studied. The findings of Rumsfeld et al. (2004) and Perski et al. (1998) add to the increasing evidence that the mental health status is linked to outcomes in cardiac patients. Mallik et al. (2005) showed that depression appeared to be a strong inverse risk factor for physical functioning. Ai et al. (1997) in turn, using depression as the outcome measure, found that depression 1 year post-CABG was predicted by somatic factors such as non-cardiac chronic illnesses, postoperative fatigue and shortness of breath.

The present study applied a cross-lagged panel design to examine whether poorer physical functioning led to a higher level of depression or – vice versa – a higher depression level predicted poorer physical functioning. Depression turned out to clearly predict physical functioning and not vice versa. The predictive priority of depression over physical functioning could be demonstrated for both time intervals of interest: from the day before surgery to the time 2 months after surgery and from 2 months to 1 year after surgery. Using the procedure of structural equation modelling, it was also possible to directly compare the strength of the above-described longitudinal paths between men and women. The strength of these paths did not differ with respect to gender, thus slightly departing from the results of other studies, which reported a stronger relationship between depression and physical functioning among women than among men (Mallik et al., 2005; Mendes de Leon et al., 1998). However, the comparability of their results is of restricted value, since neither of these studies controlled for the cross-lagged relationship, and outcome parameters in the study of Mendes de Leon et al. were cardiac events and not physical functioning.

Several mechanisms by which depression confers increased risk for heart patients have been discussed. Depression is associated with a number of behavioural risk factors, such as smoking, alcohol abuse and physical inactivity (Ladwig et al., 1999) as well as nonadherence to medications (Rieckmann et al., 2006). Possible mechanisms on a physiological level include inflammation (Carney et al., 2001) and increased platelet aggregability (Musselman et al., 1996).

The results not only confirm the close relationship between physical depression and functioning, but also emphasize the vital importance of depression within the recovery process. However, this study was observational in design and does not allow "causal" interpretation. Any causal statement should be made with great care and only within the setting of an experimental design (cf. Faller and Bulzebruck, 2002).

## 5.4 Limitations

There are some possible limitations to this study, which should be taken into account in its interpretation. Limitations concern (1) study measurements, (2) drop-out rate (3) sample size and (4) generalizability.

(1) The Patient Health Questionnaire (PHQ) is a brief screening instrument to assess depression severity. Since there is strong evidence for both high sensitivity and specificity when diagnosing major depression (Kroenke et al., 2002), this instrument seems appropriate to epidemiological questions. Nevertheless the use of the PHQ cannot replace clinical diagnosis. However, the diagnosis of major depression was not the predominant object of interest. Because it was of utmost interest to use all the information available, the original continuous variable instead of the dichotomized version was employed.

Physical functioning was assessed with the subscale of the SF-36 health survey, which is a global instrument and not as detailed as disease-specific instruments. This disadvantage may be outweighed by the fact that the SF-36 has become a standard instrument, which enhances comparability with other studies.

The housework questionnaire by Worringen et al. (2001) was applied to assess the time spent on housework and the stress through housework. Stress through housework was assessed with a single-item instrument, and there was no formal assessment of its reliability. This limitation, however, would tend to bias the study toward the null hypothesis. Despite this fact, demands were strongly associated with outcome parameters. Moreover, the household score has not been well validated yet. Specifically, the term "household" and "demands by household" could evoke different mental representations in men and women. Men could, for example, think of a multitude of single activities, whereas women might integrate the whole procedure of planning (Worringen et al., 2001).

No data was available to differentiate between cardiac mortality and all-cause mortality. However, since the primary goal of the study was to evaluate psychosocial variables, the main focus was not on clinical issues. Several studies (Blumenthal et al., 2003) did not differentiate between different causes either, so that the comparability was not reduced by this limitation.

(2) A serious limitation for the interpretation of the follow-up might be the drop-out rate in this study: though patients were approached by phone and in writing, roughly one third of the patients did not complete the questionnaires at all three measurement points. The drop-out rate was similar to that in other studies on CABG (e.g. Sjoland et al., 1999). In this study, the drop-out was confounded with central variables of interest. Therefore, the representativeness of results may be restricted. However, because the differences between the two genders in these variables were more marked in the full sample, the danger of exaggerating gender differences due to the drop-out, i.e. the danger of producing an $\alpha$-error, is limited. Moreover, great efforts were made to use all the available data. Imputation methods were applied to missing data within each cross-sectional wave instead of pairwise or listwise exclusion of missing values.

(3) Due to a relatively small sample size, the analyses were restricted in some ways. With respect to mortality, the power of the sample was too small to conduct analyses separately for men and women or to include higher interaction terms. Moreover, only approximately one fifth of the study population was female. The different sample sizes of men and women required special attention for some statistical assumptions such as homogeneity of variances. Comparing differing sample sizes also called attention to effect sizes as an indicator of strength of differences rather than to significance alone.

(4) All patients were recruited at a single centre, the Deutsches Herzzentrum Berlin (German Heart Institute Berlin). Given the high reputation of this centre, it is possible that cases that are more complicated may have been referred to this hospital and thus the study sample may represent a less healthy population. On the other hand, since it was possible to carefully adjust for a multitude of clinical factors in this study, the role of psychosocial factors can be assumed to remain largely unbiased.

## 5.5 Clinical Implications

The present study contributes towards an understanding of gender differences in mortality and physical functioning in bypass patients. This section deals with the possible clinical implications.

*(1) Independent of gender, the operation appears to be a great stressor causing high levels of anxiety and depression.* Almost every second woman and every fourth man experience a clinically relevant degree of anxiety before surgery. Moreover, a considerable proportion of both genders exhibit a high level of depression. The elevated scores can be interpreted either as a reaction to preoperative physical limitations or as stress-induced by the upcoming surgery. After surgery, these rates decline considerably. It is generally acknowledged that preoperative depression and anxiety significantly influence quality of life as well as mortality. Although the influence of psychosocial factors on physical illnesses is undisputed, the assessment of these factors is somewhat neglected in the day-to-day clinical routine (Specht et al., 2002). As a consequence, regardless of gender, depressive symptoms deserve closer psychiatric evaluation. At present, the prevalence of anxiety disorders and depression prior to surgery is vastly underestimated. Recently, efforts have been made to develop simple screening instruments, which can be integrated into patient-doctor communication despite the well-known shortage of time. For example, the Lübeck Standardized Interview for Psychosocial Screening (LIPS) (Specht et al., 2002) assesses several facets of psychosocial stress factors such as lack of social support and depression. Moreover, instruments such as the Hospital Anxiety and Depression Scale (HADS) are economic measures and have shown their excellent validity over the recent

years. With the help of such diagnostic instruments, risk patients can be identified, thus preparing the way for early psychosocial interventions.

(2) *Depression is the dominant psychosocial risk factor, less marked for mortality but stronger for subjective quality of life.* Depression is a rather heterogeneous construct, comprising a great variety of empirical conditions (e.g. Davison and Neale, 2002). Therefore the design of appropriate clinical interventions is a subtle task as can be seen from the few recent intervention studies. In the ENRICHD trial, cognitive behavioural therapy and additional optional drug treatment was effective, not only improving depression but also increasing the survival rate and reducing the recurrence of MI (Taylor, 2003). A contrasting finding was provided by the M-HART programme: offering individual interventions to patients with acute MI neither improved nor worsened the health status in men; in women, however, rates of cardiac and all-cause mortality even indicated the possibility of harm (Frasure-Smith et al., 1999). However, evidence from the M-HART programme several years later suggested that patients with short-term improvements with regard to psychological distress due to interventions had a better long-term prognosis than patients with unsuccessful outcomes in general quality of life (Cossette et al., 2001). A meta-analysis (Dusseldorp et al., 1999) that also included behaviour modification education programmes indicated that programmes, which successfully altered risk factors were most successful in reducing cardiac mortality. Finally, Callahan et al. (2005), reported an improvement in physical functioning for depressive patients by individually tailored interventions. There is still a lack of understanding of the underlying mechanisms with regard to interventions. Prior to an intervention, it is imperative to identify the precise cause of depression for each patient. For some patients who react with depressive symptoms on their foreseeing a lack of help after surgery, instrumental support may be the most appropriate intervention. For others, the use of antidepressants in particular in the initial phase of treatment may well be indicated to enhance recovery and compliance.

(3) *In the present analysis, the female subsample had a comparatively lower socioeconomic status.* This fact is probably associated with strong cohort effects and may diminish in forthcoming generations. Nonetheless, this present gender difference must be accepted as a matter of fact. Differences in living conditions appear to influence the reasons men and women give for not participating in outpatient rehabilitation programmes, such as in supervised exercise groups. Women most often give practical reasons for non-participation, citing for example that the programme is too far from their home or that they have no means of transportation. The main reasons for non-participation cited by men include a lack of interest or the opinion that the programme is "not fun" (Härtel et al., 2003). Because of this, Härtel (2005) recommends therapy

programmes that take the special circumstances of women into account. Programmes like these are based on separate female groups that deal specifically with the multiple comorbidities common to women, teach self-confidence, and provide instructions on how to make use in everyday life of what they have learned. The emphasis lies on the psychosocial and familial burdens, fears, and depression typically experienced by women. To date, such programmes have met with strong approval by female patients (Härtel, 2005). For many of the female patients self-help groups might be a valuable alternative to the conventional therapeutic interventions. A large proportion of female bypass patients lives without a partner and could profit through social support from groups of patients with the same experiences. However, sufficient data on the evaluation of the effectiveness of self-help groups are still lacking.

*(4) Women undergoing bypass surgery are on average older than men.* Some of the differences that at first glance appear to be based on gender are in reality due to age. Grande et al. (2003) have shown how age, rather than gender, determines the participation in rehabilitation measures. Focusing too narrowly on gender may easily obscure this fact. However, the overarching goal of achieving "fairness" or "equality" in health care cannot be reached by completely standardizing the services provided. Standardization carries with it the danger of neglecting the unique characteristics and needs of certain groups. The results of several studies (e.g. Grande et al., 2002; Mittag, 2002; Härtel et al., 2003) suggest that individually tailored interventions, taking into account the educational background, age and gender of each patient, will do the best in improving depression and physical functioning.

In recent years, due to the developments in medical interventions, there has been a tremendous increase in survival rates (Humphries et al., 2007). A further reduction of mortality rates may sound unrealistic, given the natural limitations through ageing processes and physical dispositions. Strong efforts should therefore aim at an enhancement of quality of life. In this domain, there is still ample space for improvements by psychosocial interventions.

## 5.6 Conclusion

Starting from the observed gender gap in early mortality rates, the present thesis had the purpose of determining, in addition to clinical factors, the role of psychosocial variables with respect to mortality and physical functioning. As for mortality, the investigation found that the gender gap could not be explained by the higher depression rates of women, but rather by the different initial status with respect to socio-economic status and age, the former serving as an indicator for a bundle of risk factors. As for physical functioning, the gender gap diminished and was then only marginal. There was not one single risk factor explaining the gender difference in physical functioning, but rather it was due to all risk factors together. The importance of depression for the recovery process could be underlined by evidence of a unidirectional relationship with physical functioning. Contrary to expectations, the recovery process turned out to be comparable between men and women, both with respect to improvement as a whole and to the correlation pattern of psychosocial variables. This implies that clinical measures to improve the situation should concentrate on the initial status. On this basis, one is naturally led to the hypothesis that clinical interventions should be tailored not predominantly to patients' gender but rather to the overall social condition. Further studies are needed to elucidate the effectiveness of interventions for groups of different social backgrounds, gender and age.

# 6 SUMMARY

The number of coronary artery bypass graft (CABG) surgeries in industrialized countries has steadily increased over the past two decades. Roughly one third of these operations are performed on women. The majority of studies on CABG operations have reported that the early mortality rate of women is roughly twice as high as that of men. A similar difference has been found with respect to the subjective health status. Studies conducted in search of an explanation of these marked gender differences have yielded conflicting results. Generally, adjustment for clinical risk factors diminished the gender gap, but did not fully explain it. So far, only few studies have paid attention to psychosocial factors. In particular, an analysis of a possible predictive relationship between depression and "physical functioning" (an indicator for the subjective health status) is missing. The purpose of this study was to determine the role of psychosocial variables in the recovery process and to examine whether gender differences in these variables, particularly in depression, explain gender differences in 1-year mortality and physical functioning. Hence, clinical variables were taken into account to adequately evaluate the contribution of psychosocial variables. Since quality of life has gained increasing importance as a patient-reported outcome parameter over recent years, the primary outcome variables were extended beyond mortality to physical functioning.

The study was part of a prospective study carried out by the Competence Network of Heart Failure (Kompetenznetz Herzinsuffizienz) funded by the German Federal Ministry of Education and Research (BMBF). It was based on a sample of 579 consecutive patients (22% women) undergoing CABG surgery at the Deutsches Herzzentrum Berlin between January 2005 and October 2005. Psychosocial factors were determined by means of questionnaires, including the Patient Health Questionnaire PHQ-9, the Hospital Anxiety and Depression Scale HADS-D, and the "social support" section from the Enhancing Recovery in Heart Patients (ENRICHD) study. Clinical data were retrieved from structured medical records and case report forms. The outcome variable physical functioning (in terms of restrictions in daily activities) was derived from the SF-36 health survey. Both psychosocial and medical data were collected at three different time points: 1 day before surgery, 2 months after surgery and 1 year after surgery. A sample of 355 patients responded at all time points.

Women operated upon were older than men ($M_{women}$ = 70.4 ± 9.3 versus $M_{men}$ = 65.3 ± 8.6), had a lower education level (25.6% of women without vocational training versus 4.6% of men) and were more likely to live alone (60.3% versus 19.0%). On average, women had a less favourable risk profile than men. Further, they showed more symptoms of depression and anxiety before CABG surgery. The 1-year mortality rate of women exceeded that of men markedly (12.4% versus 5.2%). Accordingly, women evaluated their physical functioning worse than men. It is worth noting that gender no longer remained an independent risk factor for both mortality and physical functioning after adjustment for psychosocial and clinical risk factors. Depression was the most important risk factor for both mortality (OR = 1.50, 95%CI = 1.03 - 2.19) and physical functioning ($\beta$ = -0.36) in the entire sample, but did only partially add to an explanation of the gender gap in 1-year mortality. In contrast, education level and age contributed to explaining the gender gap in mortality. Men and women differed in their baseline health status but experienced similar degrees of improvement over time. Household chores did not independently contribute to this overall process. Finally, a cross-lagged path analytic model demonstrated predictive priority of depression over physical functioning at later time points and not vice versa.

The results presented here underscore the importance of depression  - as a modifiable risk factor - for both mortality and physical functioning. In the end, possible clinical implications are discussed to some detail.

# 7 ZUSAMMENFASSUNG

Die Zahl der aortokoronaren Bypass-Operationen (CABG) ist in den vergangenen zwei Jahrzehnten in den westlichen Industriestaaten kontinuierlich gestiegen. Ungefähr 30% der Operationen werden an Frauen durchgeführt. Es besteht weitgehend Konsens, dass Frauen nach CABG eine schlechtere Prognose als Männer haben. Dies betrifft sowohl die Frühmortalitätsrate, die bei Frauen im Vergleich zu Männern um etwa das Doppelte erhöht ist, als auch einen deutlichen Geschlechterunterschied bezüglich der gesundheitsbezogenen Lebensqualität. Studien, die durchgeführt wurden, um diese markanten Geschlechterunterschiede zu erklären, haben zum Teil widersprüchliche Ergebnisse erbracht. In der Mehrzahl der Studien verringerte sich der Geschlechterunterschied durch Adjustierung mit klinischen Risikofaktoren. Diese konnten jedoch den Geschlechterunterschied nicht vollständig erklären. Nur wenige Studien haben bislang psychosoziale Faktoren berücksichtigt. Insbesondere fehlt eine Analyse des wechselseitigen Zusammenhanges zwischen Depressivität und *körperlicher Funktion* – einem Indikator für gesundheitsbezogene Lebensqualität.

Ziel dieser Studie war es, die Rolle von psychosozialen Variablen im Erholungsprozess nach CABG zu untersuchen. Von besonderem Interesse war, ob Geschlechterunterschiede bei diesen Variablen, insbesondere Depressivität, Unterschiede in der 1-Jahres-Mortalität und körperlicher Funktion erklären. Um den relativen Beitrag von psychosozialen Variablen beurteilen zu können, wurden klinische Variablen in die statistischen Auswertungen eingeschlossen. In den vergangenen Jahren hat die gesundheitsbezogene Lebensqualität deutlich an Bedeutung gewonnen. Daher ist in dieser Studie körperliche Funktion neben Mortalität der wichtigste Outcomeparameter.

Die Studie war Teil einer prospektiven Studie, die im Rahmen des vom Bundesministerium für Bildung und Forschung (BMBF) geförderten „Kompetenznetzes Herzinsuffizienz" durchgeführt wurde. Sie basierte auf einer Stichprobe von 579 konsekutiven Patienten (22% Frauen), die sich von Januar 2005 bis Oktober 2005 einer CABG-Operation am Deutschen Herzzentrum Berlin unterzogen. Psychosoziale Faktoren wurden mit Fragebögen erhoben: Depressivität mit dem „Gesundheitsfragebogen für Patienten (PHQ-D)", Angst mit der „Hospital Anxiety and Depression Scale (HADS-D)" und soziale Unterstützung mit der entsprechenden Subskala der „Enhancing Recovery in Heart Patients (ENRICHD)"-Studie. Medizinische Daten wurden den Krankenakten (Arztberichte und case report forms) entnommen. Körperliche Funktion (Beeinträchtigung der körperlichen Aktivitäten durch den Gesundheitszustand) wurde mit den SF-36 Gesundheitsfragebögen erfasst. Sowohl psychosoziale als auch medizinische Variablen wurden zu drei verschiedenen Messzeitpunkten erhoben: 1 Tag vor der Operation, 2 Monate nach der Operation und 1 Jahr nach der Operation. Die Fragebögen wurden von 355 (61.3%) der 579 Patienten zu allen drei Messzeitpunkten beantwortet.

Frauen waren im Durchschnitt älter als Männer ($M_{Frauen}$ = 70.4 ± 9.3 versus $M_{Männer}$ = 65.3 ± 8.6), hatten einen geringeren Bildungsstand (25.6% der Frauen ohne Berufsausbildung versus 4.6% der Männer) und lebten häufiger alleine (60.3% versus 19.0%). Darüber hinaus hatten Frauen ein insgesamt ungünstigeres Risikofaktorenprofil als Männer.

Die 1-Jahres-Mortalitätsrate der Frauen überstieg die der Männer deutlich (12.4% versus 5.2%). Entsprechend schlechter wurde von den Frauen auch der subjektive Gesundheitszustand eingeschätzt. Geschlecht war nach Adjustierung mit psychosozialen und klinischen Risikofaktoren weder für Mortalität noch für körperliche Funktion ein unabhängiger Prädiktor. Als wichtigster unabhängiger Risikofaktor in der Gesamtstichprobe kristallisierte sich sowohl für Mortalität (OR = 1.50, 95% CI = 1.03 - 2.19) als auch für körperliche Funktion (β = -0.36) die Depressivität heraus. Der Beitrag von Depressivität zur Aufklärung des Geschlechterunterschiedes bezüglich Mortalität und körperlicher Funktion war jedoch marginal. Dagegen mediierten Bildungsniveau und Alter den Zusammenhang zwischen Geschlecht und Outcomeparametern.

Männer und Frauen unterschieden sich in ihrem präoperativen Gesundheitsstatus, zeigten jedoch im 1-Jahresverlauf eine ähnliche Verbesserung ihres Gesundheitszustandes. Belastungen durch Hausarbeit schienen diesen Erholungsprozess insgesamt nur wenig zu beeinflussen. Abschließend konnte mit einem „cross-lagged panel design" gezeigt werden, dass in der Längsschnittanalyse Depressivität ein wichtiger determinierender Faktor für körperliche Funktion ist und nicht vice versa.

Die Ergebnisse dieser Studie unterstreichen die Bedeutung von Depressivität als Risikofaktor für Mortalität und körperliche Funktion. Die sich daraus ergebenden klinischen Implikationen werden diskutiert.

# 8 REFERENCES

## 8.1 Literature

Abramov, D., Tamariz, M. G., Sever, J. Y., Christakis, G. T., Bhatnagar, G., Heenan, A. L., et al. (2000). The influence of gender on the outcome of coronary artery bypass surgery. *The Annals of Thoracic Surgery, 70*(3), 800-805.

Ades, P. A., Waldman, M. L., Polk, D. M., & Cofolesky, J. T. (1992). Referral patterns and exercise response in the rehabilitation of female coronary patients aged greater than or equal to 62 years. *The American Journal of Cardiology, 69*, 1422-1425.

Ahrens, W., Bellach, B.M., & Jöckel, K.H. (Hrsg.) (1998) *Messung soziodemographischer Merkmale in der Epidemiologie*. RKI Schriften 1/98. Berlin: Robert Koch-Institut.

Ai, A. L., Peterson, C., Dunkle, R. E., Saunders, D. G., Bolling, S. F., & Buchtel, H. A. (1997). How gender affects psychological adjustment one year after coronary artery bypass graft surgery. *Women & Health, 26*, 45-65.

Aiken, L. S., & West, S. G. (1991). *Multiple Regression: Testing and Interpreting Interactions*. Newbury Park, CA: Sage Publications.

Albus, C., & Siegrist, J. (2005). Primärprävention—Psychosoziale Aspekte. *Zeitschrift für Kardiologie, 94*(3), III/105-III/112.

Allen, J. K., Fitzgerald, S. T., Swank, R. T., & Becker, D. M. (1990). Functional status after coronary artery bypass grafting and percutaneous transluminal coronary angioplasty. *The American Journal of Cardiology, 66*(12), 921-925.

Arbuckle, J. L. (1999). *Amos for Windows. Version 4.01*. Chicago: SmallWaters Corp.

Arbuckle, J. L., & Wottke, W. (1995). *AMOS 4.0 User's Guide*. Chicago: SmallWaters Corp.

Artinian, N. T., & Duggan, C. H. (1995). Sex differences in patient recovery patterns after coronary artery bypass surgery. *Heart & Lung, 24*, 483-494.

Barefoot, J. C., Helms, M. J., Mark, D. B., Blumenthal, J. A., Califf, R. M., Haney, T. L., et al. (1996). Depression and long-term mortality risk in patients with coronary artery disease. *The American Journal of Cardiology, 78*(6), 613-617.

Barnes, S. A., Lindborg, S. R., & Seaman, J. W. J. (2006). Multiple imputation techniques in small sample clinical trials. *Statistics in Medicine, 25*(2), 233-245.

Baron, R. M., & Kenny, D. A. (1986). The moderator-mediator variable distinction in social psychological research: conceptual, strategic, and statistical considerations. *Journal of Personality and Social Psychology, 51*(6), 1173-1182.

Barry, L. C., Kasl, S. V., Lichtman, J., Vaccarino, V., & Krumholz, H. M. (2006). Social support and change in health-related quality of life 6 months after coronary artery bypass grafting. *Journal of Psychosomatic Research, 60*, 185-193.

Berkman, L. F., & Glass, T. (2000). *Social epidemiology*. New York: Oxford University Press.

Berkman, L. F., Leo-Summer, L., & Horwitz, R. I. (1992). Emotional support and survival after myocardial infarction. A prospective, population-based study of the elderly. *Annals of Internal Medicine, 117*, 1003-1009.

Berkman, L. F., & Syme, S. L. (1979). Social networks, host resistance, and mortality: A nine-year follow-up study of Alameda county residents. *American Journal of Epidemiology, 109*(2), 186-204.

Berkman, L. F., Vaccarino, V., & Seeman, T. (1993). Gender differences in cardiovascular morbidity and mortality: The contribution of social networks and support. *Annals of Behavioral Medicine, 15*, 112-118.

Blankstein, R., Ward, R. P., Arnsdorf, M., Jones, B., Lou, Y. B., & Pine, M. (2005). Female gender is an independent predictor of operative mortality after coronary artery bypass graft surgery: contemporary analysis of 31 Midwestern hospitals. *Circulation, 112*(9 Suppl), I323-327.

Blumenthal, J. A., Lett, H. S., Babyak, M. A., White, W., Smith, P. K., Mark, D. B., et al. (2003). Depression as a risk factor for mortality after coronary artery bypass surgery. *The Lancet, 362*, 604-609.

Boogard, M. A. K., & Broidy, M. E. (1985). Comparsion of the rehabilitation of men and women post- myocardinal infarction. *Journal of Cardiopulmonary Rehabilitation, 5*, 379-384.

Borowicz, L. J., Royall, R., Grega, M., Selnes, O., Lyketsos, C., & McKhann, G. (2002). Depression and cardiac morbidity 5 years after coronary artery bypass surgery. *Psychosomatics, 43*(6), 464-471.

Brandrup-Wognsen, G., Berggren, H., Hartford, M., Hjalmarson, A., Karlsson, T., & Herlitz, J. (1996). Female sex is associated with increased mortality and morbidity early, but not late, after coronary artery bypass grafting. *European Heart Journal, 17*(9), 1426-1431.

Bresser, P. J., Sexton, D. L., & Foell, D. W. (1993). Patient's response to postpronement of coronary artery bypass graft surgery. *Journal of Nursery Scholarship, 25*(1), 5-10.

Brezinka, V., & Kittel, F. (1996). Psycosocial factors of coronary heart disease in women: a review. *Social Science & Medicine, 42*, 1351-1365.

Brezinka, V., Maes, S. & Dusseldorp, E. (2001). Gender differences in psychological impairment after a coronary incident. *Personality and Individual Differences, 30*, 127-135.

Bullinger, M., & Kirchberger, I. ( 1998). *SF-36 Fragebogen zum Gesundheitszustand - Handanweisung*. Göttingen: Hogrefe.

Burg, M. M., Benedetto, M. C., Rosenberg, R., & Soufer, R. (2003). Presurgical depression predicts medical morbidity 6 months after coronary artery bypass graft surgery. *Psychosomatic Medicine, 66*(1), 111-118.

Bute, B. P., Mathew, J., Blumenthal, J. A., James, A., Welsh-Bohmer, K., White, W., et al. (2003). Female gender is associated with impaired quality of life 1 year after coronary artery bypass surgery. *Psychosomatic Medicine, 65*(6), 944-951.

Callahan, C. M., Kroenke, K., Counsell, S. R., Hendrie, H. C., Perkins, A. J., Katon, W., et al. (2005). Treatment of depression improves physical functioning in older adults. *Journal of the American Geriatrics Society, 53*(3), 367-373.

Carney, R. M., Blumenthal, J. A., Stein, P. K., Watkins, L., Catellier, D., Berkman, L. F., et al. (2001). Depression, heart rate variability, and acute myocardial infarction. *Circulation, 104*(17), 2024-2028.

Connerney, I., Shapiro, P. A., & McLaughlin, J. S. (2001). Relation between depression after coronary artery bypass surgery and 12-month outcome: A prospective study. *The Lancet, 358*, 1766-1771.

Cossette, S., Frasure-Smith, N., & Lesperance, F. (2001). Clinical implications of a reduction in psychological distress on cardiac prognosis in patients participating in a psychosocial intervention program. *Psychosomatic Medicine, 63*(2), 257-266.

Davison, G. C., & Neale, J. M. (2002). *Klinische Psychologie. Ein Lehrbuch* (6th ed.). Weinheim: Beltz PVU.

Duits, A. A., Boeke, S., Taams, M. A., Passchier, J., & Erdman, R. A. M. (1997). Prediction of quality of life after coronary artery bypass graft surgery: a review and evaluation of multiple, recent studies. *Psychosomatic Medicine, 59*, 257-268.

Dusseldorp, E., van Elderen, T., Maes, S., Meulman, J., & Kraaij, V. (1999). A meta-analysis of psychoeduational programs for coronary heart disease patients. *Health Psychology, 18*(5), 506-519.

Eagle, K. A., Guyton, R. A., & Davidoff, R. (1999). American College of Cardiology/American Heart Association ACC/AHA Guidelines for Coronary Artery Bypass Graft Surgery: A Report of the American College of Cardiology/American Heart Association Task Force on Practice Guidelines (Committee to Revise the 1991 Guidelines for Coronary Artery Bypass Graft Surgery). *Journal of the American College of Cardiology, 34*, 1262-1347.

Edwards, A. C., Nazroo, J. Y., & Brown, G. W. (1998). Gender differences in marital support following a shared life event. *Social Science & Medicine, 46*(8), 1077-1085.

Edwards, F. H., Carey, J. S., Grover, F. L., Bero, J. W., & Hartz, R. S. (1998). Impact of gender on coronary bypass operative mortality. *The Annals of Thoracic Surgery, 66*(1), 125.

Elizur, Y., & Hirsh, E. (1999). Psychosocial adjustment and mental health two months after coronary artery bypass surgery: a multisystemic analysis of patients' resources. *Journal of Behavioral Medicine, 22*(2), 157-177.

Emery, C. F., Frid, D. J., Engebretson, T. O., Alonzo, A. A., Fish, A., Ferketich, A. K., et al. (2004). Gender differences in quality of life among cardiac patients. *Psychosomatic Medicine, 66*(2), 190-197.

Ensel, W. M. (1986). Sex, marital status, and depression: The role of life events and social support. In N. Lin, A. Dean & W. M. Ensel (Eds.), *Social support, life events, and depression* (pp. 231-247). Orlando, FL: Academic Press.

Faller, H., & Bulzebruck, H. (2002). Coping and survival in lung cancer: a 10-year follow-up. *American Journal of Psychiatry, 159*(12), 2105-2107.

Faller, H., Schilling, S., & Lang, H. (1994). Verbessert Coping das Befinden? Ergebnisse einer Längsschnittuntersuchung mit Bronchialkarzinompatienten (Does coping improve emotional adjustment? Results of a longitudinal study with bronchial carcinoma patients). *Psychotherapie, Psychosomatik, Medizinische Psychologie, 44*(9-10), 355-364.

Frasure-Smith, N., Lesperance, F., Juneau, M., Talajic, M., & Bourassa, M. G. (1999). Gender, depression, and one-year prognosis after myocardial infarction. *Psychosomatic Medicine, 61*, 26-37.

Ghali, W. A., Quan, H., Shrive, F. M., & Hirsch, G. M. (2003). Outcomes after coronary artery bypass graft surgery in Canada: 1992/93 to 2000/01. *The Canadian Journal of Cardiology, 19*(7), 774-781.

Grande, G., Leppin, A., Mannebach, H., Romppel, M., & Altenhöner, T. H. (2002). *Geschlechtsspezifische Unterschiede in der kardiologischen Rehabilitation: Abschlussbericht.* Bielefeld: Universität Bielefeld.

Haffner, S. M., Katz, M. S., & Dunn, J. F. (1991). Increased upper body and overall adiposity is associated with decreased sex hormone binding globulin in postmenopausal women. *International Journal of Obesity, 15*(7), 471-478.

Hansen, E. F., Andersen, L. T., & von Eyben, F. E. (1993). Cigarette smoking and age at first acute myocardial infarction and influence of gender and extent of smoking. *The American Journal of Cardiology, 71*, 1439-1442.

Härtel, U. (2003). *Ist-Analyse Prävalenz der Herz-Kreislauferkrankungen bei Frauen in NRW. Gutachten im Auftrag der Enquete-Kommission "Zukunft einer frauengerechten Gesundheitsversorgung in NRW".* Düsseldorf. Online available: www.landtag.nrw.de/portal/WWW/GB_I/I.1/ EK/EKALT/13_EK2/aktuelles.jsp [30.07.07].

Härtel, U. (2005). Geschlechtsspezifische Unterschiede in der kardiologischen Rehabilitation. *Informiert!,9*, 11-12.

Härtel, U., Gehring, J., Klein, G., & Symannek, C. (2003). *Untersuchung geschlechtsspezifischer, biomedizinischer und psychosozialer Einflüsse auf den langfristigen Erfolg von Reha-Maßnahmen bei Patienten mit koronarer Herzkrankheit*: Abschlussbericht (1. Förderphase) BMBF Bericht.

Helgeson, V. S. (2005). *The psychology of gender* (2nd ed.). New Jersey: Pearson Education Inc.

Herrmann C., Buss U., & Snaith R.P. (1995) *HADS-D. Hospital Anxiety and Depression Scale-Deutsche Version.* Bern: Hans Huber.

Helgeson, V. S., & Fritz, H. L. (1996). Implications of communication and unmitigated communication for adolescent adjustment to type 1 diabetes. *Women's Health: Research on Gender, Behavior, and Policy, 2*(3), 169-194.

Hobfoll, S. E., & Schumm, J. A. (2004). Die Theorie der Ressourcenerhaltung: Anwendung auf die öffentliche Gesundheitsförderung. In P. Buchwald, C. Schwarzer & S. E. Hobfoll (Eds.), *Stress gemeinsam bewältigen* (pp. 91-120). Göttingen: Hogrefe.

Hobfoll, S. E., & Wells, J. D. (1998). Conservation of resources, stress, and aging: Why do some slide and some spring? In J. Lomranz (Ed.), *Handbook of Aging and Mental Health: An Integrative Approach* (pp.121-134). New York: Springer.

House, J. S., Robbins, C., & Metzner, H. L. (1982). The association of social relationships and activities with mortality: prospective evidence from the Tecumseh Community Health Study. *American Journal of Epidemiology, 116*(1), 123-140.

Humphries, K. H., Gao, M., Pu, A., Lichtenstein, S., & Thompson, C. R. (2007). Significant improvement in short-term mortality in women undergoing coronary artery bypass surgery (1991 to 2004). *Journal of the American College of Cardiology, 49*(14), 1552-1558.

Hunt, J. O., Hendrata, M. V., & Myls, P. (2000). Quality of life 12 months after coronary artery bypass graft surgery. *Heart & Lung, 29*(6), 401-411.

Jenson, M., Suls, J., & Lemos, K. (2003). A comparison of physical activity in men and women with cardiac disease: do gender roles complicate recovery? *Women & Health, 37*(1), 31-47.

Jiang, L., Tsubakihara, M., Heinke, M. Y., Yao, M., Dunn, M. J., Phillips, W., et al. (2001). Heart failure and apoptosis: electrophoretic methods support data from micro- and macro-arrays. A critical review of genomics and proteomics. *Proteomics, 1*(12), 1481-1488.

Jousilahti, P., Vartiainen, E., Tuomilehto, J., & Puska, P. (1996). Twenty-year dynamics of serum cholesterol levels in the middle-aged population of eastern Finland. *Annals of Internal Medicine, 125*(9), 713-722.

Kaltenbach, M., & Olbrich, H. G. (2000). Herzinsuffizienz. In M. Kaltenbach (Ed.), *Kardiologie kompakt* (pp. 319-330). Darmstadt: Steinkopff.

Kannel, W. B. (2000). Incidence and epidemiology of heart failure. *Heart Failure Review, 5*(2), 167-173.

Kannel, W. B., & Wilson, P. W. (1995). Risk factors that attenuate the female coronary disease advantage. *Archives of Internal Medicine, 155*(1), 57-61.

King, K. B., Porter, L. A., & Rowe, M. A. (1994). Functional, social, and emotional outcomes in women and men in the first year following coronary artery bypass surgery. *Journal of Women's Health, 3*, 347-354.

King, K. B., Reis, H. T., Porter, L. A., & Norsen, L. H. (1993). Social support and long-term recovery from coronary artery surgery: effects on patients and spouses. *Health Psychology, 12*(1), 56-63.

King, K. M. (2000). Gender and short-term recovery from cardiac surgery. *Nursing Research, 49*, 29-36.

Knoll, N., Scholz, U., & Rieckmann, N. (2005). *Einführung in die Gesundheitspsychologie*. München: Ernst Reinhardt Verlag/UTB.

Koivula, M., Paunonen-Ilmonen, M., Tarkka, M.-T., Tarkka, M., & Laippala, P. (2001). Gender differences and fears in patients awaiting coronary artery bypass. *Journal of Clinical Nursing, 10*, 538-549.

Kroenke, K., Spitzer, R. L., & Williams, J. B. W. (2002). The PHQ-15: validity of a new measure for evaluating the severity of somatic symptoms. *Psychosomatic Medicine, 64*(2), 258-266.

Kulik, J. A., & Mahler, H. I. M. (1989). Social support and recovery from surgery. *Health Psychology, 8*, 221-238.

Lacey, E. A., & Walters, S. J. (2003). Continuing inequality: gender and social class influences on self perceived health after a heart attack. *Journal of Epidemiology and Community Health, 57*(8), 622-627.

Ladwig, K.-H., Erazo, N., & Rugulies, R. (2004). *Depression, Angst und vitale Erschöpfung vor Ausbruch der koronaren Herzkrankheit*. Frankfurt a. M.: VAS-Verlag für akademische Schriften.

Laireiter, A., & Baumann, U. (1992). Network structures and support functions: Theoretical and empirical analyses. In H. O. F. Veiel & U. Baumann (Eds.), *The meaning and measurement of social support* (pp. 33-55). Washington, DC: Hemisphere.

Langeluddecke, P., Fulcher, G., & Baird, D. (1989). A prospective evaluation of the psychosocial effects of coronary artery bypass surgery. *Journal of Psychosomatic Research, 33*, 37-45.

LaRosa, J. C., Hunninghake, D., Bush, D., Criqui, M. H., Getz, G. S., Gotto, A. M., Jr., et al. (1990). The cholesterol facts. A summary of the evidence relating dietary fats, serum cholesterol, and coronary heart disease. A joint statement by the American Heart Association and the National Heart, Lung, and Blood Institute. The Task Force on Cholesterol Issues, American Heart Association. *Circulation, 81*(5), 1721-1733.

Lee, G. R., Willetts, M. C., & Seccombe, K. (1998). Widowhood and depression: Gender differences. *Research on Aging, 20*, 611-630.

Lemos, K., Suls, J., Jenson, M., Lounsbury, P., & Gordon, E. E. I. (2003). How do female and male cardiac patients and their spouses share responsibilities after discharge from the hospital? *Annals of Behavioral Medicine, 25*, 8-15.

Löwe, B., Spitzer, R. L., Grafe, K., Kroenke, K., Quenter, A., Zipfel, S., et al. (2004). Comparative validity of three screening questionnaires for DSM-IV depressive disorders and physicians' diagnoses. *Journal of Affective Disorders, 78*(2), 131-140.

Löwe, B., Spitzer, R. L., Zipfel, S., & Herzog, W. (2002). *Patient Health Questionnaire (PHQ), German Version, Manual and Materials* (2nd ed.). Karlsruhe: Pfizer.

Löwel, H., Döring, A., Schneider, A., Heier, M., Thorand, B., & Meisinger, C. (2005). The MONICA Augsburg surveys - basis for prospective cohort studies. *Gesundheitswesen, 67 Suppl 1*, 13-18.

Löwel, H., Koenig, W., Engel, S., Hormann, A., & Keil, U. (2000). The impact of diabetes mellitus on survival after myocardial infarction: can it be modified by drug treatment? Result of a population-based myocardial infarction register follow-up study. *Diabetologia, 43*, 218-226.

Löwel, H., Lewis, M., Keil, U., Hörmann, A., Bolte, H. D., Willich, S., et al. (1995). Zeitliche Trends von Herzinfarktmorbidität, -mortalität, 28-Tage-Letalität und medizinischer Versorgung. Ergebnisse des Augsburger Herzinfarktregisters von 1985 bis 1992. *Zeitschrift für Kardiologie, 84*, 596-605.Löwel, H., Stieber, J., Koenig, W., Thorand, B., Hörmann, A., Gostomzyk, J., et al. (1999). Das Diabetes-bedingte Herzinfarktrisiko in einer süddeutschen Bevölkerung. Ergebnisse der MONICA-Augsburg Studien 1985-1995. *Diabetologie und Stoffwechsel, 8*, 11-21.

Lund, R., Due, P., Modvig, J., Holstein, B. E., Damsgaard, M. T., & Andersen, P. K. (2002). Cohabitation and marital status as predictors of mortality: An eight year follow-up study. *Social Science & Medicine, 55*, 673-679.

Mallik, S., Krumholz, H. M., Lin, Z. Q., Kasl, S. V., Mattera, J., Roumains, S., et al. (2005). Patients with depressive symptoms have lower health status benefits after coronary artery bypass surgery. *Circulation, 111*, 271-277.

Mayou, R., & Bryant, B. (1987). Quality of life after coronary artery surgery. *The Quarterly Journal of Medicine, 62*(239), 239-248.

McKhann, G. M., Borowitz, L. M., Goldsborough, M. A., Enger, C., & Sclncs, O. A. (1997). Depression and cognitive decline after coronary artery bypass grafting. *The Lancet, 349*, 1282-1284.

Mendes de Leon, C. F., Krumholz, H. M., Seeeman, T. S., Vaccarino, V., Williams, C. S., Kasl, S. V., et al. (1998). Depression and risk of coronary heart disease in elderly men and women: New Haven EPESE, 1982-1991. Established Poulations for the Epdemiologic Studies of the Elderly. *Archives of Internal Medicine, 158*, 2341-2348.

Mitchell, R. H., Robertson, E., Harvey, P. J., Nolan, R., Rodin, G., Romans, S., et al. (2005). Sex differences in depression after coronary artery bypass graft surgery. *American Heart Journal, 150*(5), 1017-1025.

Mittag, O. (2002). *Vergleich der Verläufe nach erstem Herzinfarkt bzw. ACVB-Operation oder PTCA bei Frauen und Männern*: B-1 Projekt im Norddeutschen Forschungsverbund. Abschlussbericht 1. Förderphase.

Moore, S. M. (1995). A comparison of women's and men's symptoms during home recovery after coronary artery bypass surgery. *Heart & Lung, 24*, 495-501.

Mosca, L., Manson, J. E., Sutherland, S. E., Langer, R. D., Manolio, T., & Barrett-Connor, E. (1997). Cardiovascular disease in women: a statement for healthcare professionals from the American Heart Association. Writing Group. *Circulation, 96*(7), 2468-2482.

Musselman, D. L., Tomer, A., Manatunga, A. K., Knight, B. T., Porter, M. R., Kasey, S., et al. (1996). Exaggerated platelet reactivity in major depression. *American Journal of Psychiatry, 153*, 1313-1317.

Myrtek, M. (2001). Meta-analyses of prospective studies on coronary heart disease, type A personality, and hostility. *International Journal of Cardiology, 79*, 245-251.

Nashef, S. A. M., Roques, F., Michel, P., Gauducheau, E., Lemeshow, S., & Salamon, R. (1999). European system for cardiac operative risk evaluation (EuroSCORE). *European Journal of Cardio-Thoracic Surgery, 16*(1), 9.

Nolen-Hoeksema, S. (2001). Gender differences in depression. *Current Directions in Psychological Science, 10*(5), 173-176.

O'Rourke, D. J., Malenka, D. J., Olmstead, E. M., Quinton, H. B., Sanders, J. H., Jr., Lahey, S. J., et al. (2001). Improved in-hospital mortality in women undergoing coronary artery bypass grafting. Northern New England Cardiovascular Disease Study Group. *The Annals of Thoracic Surgery, 71*(2), 507-511.

Orth-Gomer, K., Wamala, S. P., Horsten, M., Schenck-Gustafsson, K., Schneiderman, N., & Mittleman, M. A. (2000). Marital stress worsens prognosis in women with coronary heart disease: The Stockholm Female Coronary Risk Study. *Journal of the American Medical Association, 284*, 3008-3014.

Osswald, B. R., Tochtermann, U., Schweiger, P., Thomas, G., Vahl, C. F., & Hagl, S. (2001). Does the completeness of revascularization contribute to an improved early survival in patients up to 70 years of age? *Journal of Thoracic and Cardiovascular Surgery, 49*(6), 373-377.

Oxman, T. E., & Hull, J. G. (1997). Social support, depression, and activities of daily living in older heart surgery patients. *The Journals of Gerontology, Series B, Psychological Sciences and Social Sciences, 52*(1), 1-14.

Park, Y. W., Zhu, S., Palaniappan, L., Heshka, S., Carnethon, M. R., & Heymsfield, S. B. (2003). The metabolic syndrome: prevalence and associated risk factor findings in the US population from the Third National Health and Nutrition Examination Survey, 1988-1994. *Archives of Internal Medicine, 163*(4), 427-436.

Perski, A., Feleke, E., Anderson, G., Samad, B. A., Westerlund, H., Ericsson, C. G., et al. (1998). Emotional distress before coronary bypass grafting limits the benefits of surgery. *American Heart Journal, 136*(3), 510-517.

Prescott, E., Hippe, M., & Schnohr, P. (1998). Smoking and risk of myocardial infarction in women and men: Longitudinal population study. *The British Medical Journal, 316*, 1043-1047.

Pugliesi, K., & Shook, S. L. (1998). Gender, ethnicity, and network characteristics: Variation in social support resources. *Sex Roles, 38*, 215-238.

Regitz-Zagrosek, V., Lehmkuhl, E., Hocher, B., Goesmann, D., Lehmkuhl, H. B., Hausmann, H., et al. (2004). Gender as a risk factor in young, not in old, women undergoing coronary artery bypass grafting. *Journal of the American College of Cardiology, 44*(11), 2413-2414.

Regitz-Zagrosek, V., Lehmkuhl, E., & Weickert, M. O. (2006). Gender differences in the metabolic syndrome and their role for cardiovascular disease. *Clinical Research in Cardiology, 95*(3), 136-147.

Rexrode, K. M., Buring, J. E., & Manson, J. E. (2001). Abdominal and total adiposity and risk of coronary heart disease in men. *International Journal of Obesity and Related Metabolic Disorders, 25*(7), 1047-1056.

Rexrode, K. M., Manson, J. E., & Hennekens, C. H. (1996). Obesity and cardiovascular disease. *Current Opinion in Cardiology, 11*(5), 490-495.

Rich-Edwards, J. W., Manson, J. E., Hennekens, C. H., & Buring, J. E. (1995). The primary prevention of coronary heart disease in women. *New England Journal of Medicine, 332*(26), 1758-1766.

Rieckmann, N. (2003). *Anpassung und Resilienz bei mittelalten, jungen alten und alten Kataraktpatienten.* Unpublished Dissertation, Freie Universität, Berlin. Online available: www.diss.fu-berlin.de/2003/225 [30.07.07]

Rieckmann, N., Gerin, W., Kronish, I. M., Burg, M. M., Chaplin, W. F., Kong, G., et al. (2006). Course of Depressive Symptoms and Medication Adherence After Acute Coronary Syndromes: An Electronic Medication Monitoring Study. *Journal of the American College of Cardiology, 48*(11), 2218.

Roques, F., Nashef, S. A. M., Michel, P., Pinna Pintor, P., David, M., Baudet, E., et al. (2000). Does EuroSCORE work in individual European countries? *European Journal of Cardio-Thoracic Surgery, 18*(1), 27.

Rose, G. L., Suls, J., & Green, P. J. (1996). Comparison of adjustment, activity, and tangible social support in men and women patients and their spouses during the six months post-myocardial infarction. *Annals Of Behavioral Medicine, 18*, 264-272.

Ross, C. E. (1995). Reconceptualizing marital status as a continuum of social attachment. *Journal of Marriage and the Family, 57*, 129-140.

Ross, C. E., & Mirowsky, J. (1990). The impact of the family on health: The decade in review. *Journal of Marriage and the Family, 52*, 1059-1078.

Rumsfeld, J. S., Ho, P. M., Magid, D. J., McCarthy, M., Jr., Shroyer, A. L., MaWhinney, S., et al. (2004). Predictors of health-related quality of life after coronary artery bypass surgery. *The Annals of Thoracic Surgery, 77*(5), 1508-1513.

Saur, C. D., Granger, B. B., Muhlbaier, L. H., Forman, L. M., McKenzie, R. J., Taylor, M. C., et al. (2001). Depressive symptoms and outcome of coronary artery bypass grafting. *American Journal of Critical Care, 10*(1), 4-10.

Schafer, J. L. (1999). Multiple imputation: a primer. *Statistical Methods of Medical Research, 8*(1), 3-15.

Schwarzer, R., & Rieckmann, N. (2002). Social support, cardiovascular disease, and mortality. In G. Weidner, M. S. Kopp & M. Kristenson (Eds.), *Heart disease: environment, stress and gender* (pp. 185-194). Amsterdam: IOS Press.

Shye, D., Mullooly, J. P., Freeborn, D. K., & Pope, C. R. (1995). Gender differences in the relationship between social network support and mortality: a longitudinal study of an elderly cohort. *Social Science & Medicine, 41*(7), 935-947.

Siegel, J. M., & Kuykendall, D. H. (1990). Loss, widowhood, and psychological distress among the elderly. *Journal of Consulting and Clinical Psychology, 58*, 519-524.

Sieverding, M. (1995). Die Gesundheit von Müttern - Ein Forschungsüberblick. *Zeitschrift für Medizinische Psychologie, 4*, 6-16.

Sjoland, H., Wiklund, I., Caidahl, K., Hartford, M., Karlsson, T., & Herlitz, J. (1999). Improvement in quality of life differs between women and men after coronary artery bypass surgery. *Journal of Internal Medicine, 245*(5), 445-454.

Specht, T., Benninghoven, D., Jantschek, G., Ebeling, A., Friedrich, S., Kunzendorf, S., et al. (2002). Psychosocial screening in coronary heart disease: 5 decisive questions. *Zeitschrift für Kardiologie, 91*(6), 458-465.

Spitzer, R. L., Kroenke, K., & Williams, J. B. W. (1999). Validation and utility of a self-report version of PRIME-MD: The PHQ primary care study. Primary Care Evaluation of Mental Disorders. Patient Health Questionnaire. *JAMA, 282*(18), 1737-1744.

Stack, S. (1998). Marriage, family, and loneliness: A cross-national study. *Sociological Perspectives, 41*(2), 415-432.

Statistisches Bundesamt. (2007). *Krankenhausstatistik (DRG-Statistik) 2005.* Wiesbaden: Statistisches Bundesamt.

Stone, R. (1999). Stress: The invisible hand in eastern Europe's death rates. In United Nations, *World Population Prospects: The 1998 Revision.*

Stroebe, M. S., & Stroebe, W. (1983). Who suffers more? Sex differences in health risks of the widowed. *Psychological Bulletin, 93*, 279-301.

Tabachnick, B. G., & Fidell, S. F. (2007). *Using Multivariate Statistics* (5th ed.). Boston: Allyn and Bacon.

Taylor, F. C., Ascione, R., Rees, K., Narayan, P., & Angelini, G. D. (2003). Socioeconomic deprivation is a predictor of poor postoperative cardiovascular outcomes in patients undergoing coronary artery bypass grafting. *Heart, 89*(9), 1062-1066.

Toumpoulis, I. K., Anagnostopoulos, C. E., Balaram, S. K., Rokkas, C. K., Swistel, D. G., Ashton, R. C., et al. (2006). Assessment of independent predictors for long-term mortality between women and men after coronary artery bypass grafting: Are women different from men? *The Journal of Thoracic and Cardiovascular Surgery, 131*, 343-351.

Tower, R. B., & Kasl, S. V. (1996). Gender, marital closeness, and depressive symptoms in elderly couples. *The Journals of Gerontology, Series B, Psychological Sciences and Social Science. 51*(3), 115-129.

Tucker, J. S., Schwartz, J. E., Clark, K. M., & Friedmann, H. S. (1999). Age-related changes in the associations of social network ties with mortality risk. *Psychology and Aging, 14*, 564-571.

Umberson, D., Wortman, C. B., & Kessler, R. C. (1992). Widowhood and depression: Explaining long-term gender differences in vulnerability. *Journal of Health and Social Behavior, 33*, 10-24.

Underwood, M. J., Firmin, R. K., & Jehu, D. (1993). Aspects of psychological and social morbidity in patients awaiting coronary artery bypass grafting. *British Heart Journal, 69*(5), 382-384.

Vaccarino, V., Abramson, J. L., Veledar, E., & Weintraub, W. S. (2002). Sex differences in hospital mortality after coronary artery bypass surgery. *Circulation, 105*, 1176-1181.

Vaccarino, V., Lin, Z. Q., Kasl, S. V., Mattera, J. A., Roumanis, S. A., Abramson, J. L. & Krumholz, H. M. (2003). Gender differences in recovery after coronary artery bypass surgery. *Journal of the American College of Cardiology, 41*, 307-314.

Vaglio, J., Jr., Conard, M., Poston, W. S., O'Keefe, J., Haddock, C. K., House, J., et al. (2004). Testing the performance of the ENRICHD Social Support Instrument in cardiac patients. *Health and Quality of Life Outcomes, 2*, 24.

van Grootheest, D. S., Beekman, A. T. F., van Groenou, M. I. B., & Deeg, D. J. H. (1999). Sex differences in depression after widowhood: Do men suffer more? *Social Psychiatry and Psychiatric Epidemiology, 34*, 391-398.

Walsh, J. M., & Grady, D. (1995). Treatment of hyperlipidemia in women. *Jama, 274*(14), 1152-1158.

Wamala, S. P., Mittleman, M. A., Horsten, M., Schenck-Gustafsson, K., & Orth-Gomer, K. (2000). Job stress and the occupational gradient in coronary heart disease risk in women. The Stockholm Female Coronary Risk Study. *Social Science & Medicine, 51*, 481-489.

Ware, J. E., Snow, K. K., & Kosinski, M. (1993). *SF-36 health survey manual and interpretation guide*. Boston (Massachuset): The Health Institute, New England Medical Center.

Weidemann, H., Meyer, K., Fischer, T., & Wetzel, A. (2003). *Frauen und koronare Herzkrankheit. Altersverteilung, Rauchen und orale Kontrazeption, klassische Rsisikofaktoren, psychosoziale Konstellationen, körperliches Training*. Frankfurt a. M..

Weissman, M. M., Bland, R. C., Canino, G. J., Faravelli, C., & Greenwald, S. (1996). Cross-national epidemiology of major depression and bipolar disorder. *JAMA, 276*, 293-299.

Wilke, N. A., Sheldahl, L. M., Dougherty, S. M., Hanna, R. D., Nickele, G. A., & Tristani, F. E. (1995). Energy expenditure during household tasks in women with coronary artery disease. *The American Journal of Cardiology, 75*(10), 670-674.

Williams, S. A., Kasl, S. V., Heiat, A., Abramson, J. L., Krumholz, H. M., & Vaccarino, V. (2002). Depression and risk of coronary heart disease among the elderly: a prospective community-based study. *Psychosomatic Medicine, 64*(1), 6-12.

Wilson, P. W., D'Agostino, R. B., Levy, D., Belanger, A. M., Silbershatz, H., & Kannel, W. B. (1998). Prediction of coronary heart disease using risk factor categories. *Circulation, 97*(18), 1837-1847.

Winkleby, M. A., Fortmann, S. P., & Barett, D. C. (1990). Social class disparities in risk factors for disease: eight-year prevalence patterns by level of education. *Preventive Medicine, 19*, 1-12.

Worringen, U., Benecke, A., Gerlich, C., & Frank, S. (2001). Erfassung von Haus- und Familienarbeit in der Rehabilitationsforschung. In U. Worringen & C. Zwingmann (Eds.), *Rehabilitation weiblich-männlich. Geschlechtsspezifische Rehabilitationsforschung* (pp. 221-234). Weinheim: Juventa.

Yusuf, S., Hawken, S., Ounpuu, S., Dans, T., Avezum, A., Lanas, F., et al. (2004). Effect of potentially modifiable risk factors associated with myocardial infarction in 52 countries (the INTERHEART study): case-control study. *The Lancet, 364*(9438), 937-952.

Zigmond, A. S., & Snaith, R. P. (1983). The hospital anxiety and depression scale. *Acta Psychiatrica Scandinavica, 67*(6), 361-370.

Zöller, B. (1999). Das Herz der Frau. *Cardio News, 2*, 12-15.

## 8.2  Tables

## 8.3 Figures

# APPENDIX

## Acknowledgements

This work was started while Professor Peter Rosemeier was still among us. With his confidence in unusual life paths, he made this work possible and generously shared his fascination of Medical Psychology as an interdisciplinary endeavour.

I am also very grateful to Professor Vera Regitz-Zagrosek. I had the privilege to profit from her broad scientific knowledge, which ranges from basic research to clinical application. Her unbiased approach to gender questions and steady support was a source of great encouragement for this work.

Data were collected at Deutsches Herzzentrum Berlin. In this context I wish to thank Professor Roland Hetzer for his ongoing interest in gender studies. My colleagues Dr. Elke Lehmkuhl and Dr. Beate Jurmann from the Heart Institute were of invaluable help in the data collection and contributed greatly with their medical expertise. Thanks go also to Anne Gale for copy-editing the manuscript.

Several wonderful colleagues and friends have contributed to this thesis by stimulating discussions and valuable ideas: Birgit Babitsch, Silke Burkert, Rolf Kienle, Nina Knoll, Ilona Oestreich, Petra Stephan, and Julia von Thienen. Brigitte Hoffmann was extremely helpful in many critical situations.

Last, but not least, I wish to thank my family for their loving support. My warmest thanks for their patience go to Justus Schmidt-Ott and to Cora and Tabea, my – sometimes critical, sometimes ironical – but always caring daughters.

Druck: Krips bv, Meppel, Niederlande
Verarbeitung: Stürtz, Würzburg, Deutschland